Effective Hospital-Physician Relationships

Effective Hospital- Physician Relationships

Stephen M. Shortell

A study conducted by the Hospital Research and Educational Trust with the support of the Estes Park Institute and the American Hospital Association's Division of Medical Affairs

Health Administration Press Perspectives
Ann Arbor, Michigan

95 94 93 92 91 90   5 4 3 2 1

Library of Congress Cataloging-in-Publication Data

Shortell, Stephen M. (Stephen Michael), date.
   Effective hospital-physician relationships / Stephen M. Shortell.
      p.   cm.
   "A study conducted by the Hospital Research and Educational Trust."
   Includes bibliographical references and index.
   ISBN 0-910701-63-6 (soft bound : acid free)
   1. Hospital-physician relations.   2. Hospital-physician relations—United States—Case studies.   I. Hospital Research and Educational Trust.   II. Title.
RA971.9.S46   1990
362.1'1'0683—dc20   90–5106

Health Administration Press
A division of the Foundation of the
   American College of Healthcare Executives
1021 East Huron Street
Ann Arbor, Michigan 48104-9990
(313) 764-1380

Hospital Research and Educational Trust
840 North Lake Shore Drive
Chicago, Illinois 60611

Estes Park Institute
P.O. Box 400
Englewood, Colorado 80151

Contents

Foreword I

Experts agree that a key characteristic of successful health care institutions is effective working relationships with physicians. Meaningful physician participation in institutional decisions on quality of care and credentialing has traditionally been the focus for physician involvement in most hospitals. The ten institutions studied in this project, however, have missions, cultures, and policies that fully integrate physicians into all phases of institutional management and governance activities. The observations and advice here are "real world" and demonstrate that good, basic communication is *the* most essential ingredient in productive working relationships.

This book is the product of a collaborative effort involving the Hospital Research and Educational Trust, the American Hospital Association's Division of Medical Affairs, and the Estes Park Institute. We offer our thanks to the ten institutions that served as the case studies for the project.

The Hospital Research and Educational Trust exists to assist hospitals and the communities they serve to improve the efficiency, quality, and accessibility of health care services. We do this by conducting applied research and demonstration projects and interpretive studies, and disseminating the results through education, publications, and other media. Hospital-physician relationships are one of five priority research areas for the Trust. We are very pleased to have contributed to this important work, and we hope that you will find this book useful.

Daniel R. Longo, Sc.D.
President
Hospital Research and
Educational Trust

Foreword II

There is nothing more important to the successful operation of a hospital than a medical staff that works in harmony with the hospital. And there is nothing more difficult to attain and to maintain. The purpose of the joint project of the Estes Park Institute, the Hospital Research and Educational Trust, and the American Hospital Association (of which this book is a result) was to explain the factors that produce such harmony where it seems to exist.

There is no magic to maintaining medical staff harmony and what this text shows is that it requires attention to detail and constant hard work. It also shows that there are very few major innovative techniques for working with the traditional medical staff. That this is so is not surprising, for the very concept of medical staff organization is inherently problematic. Thus, what is needed is constant repair to the structure, like a patient carpenter who finds the building continually falling down around him. Unfortunately, somewhat like the houses in the Marina District of San Francisco during the recent earthquake, the medical staff is built on a structure and a concept that is deeply flawed.

Yet the hospitals discussed here deserve approval and emulation, for they are finding many ways to maintain a harmonious working relationship with the physicians who are essential to them. This study's success is in the details, not in a brave new concept. And the hospitals studied are those who show that goodwill and thought can keep the relationship intact and moving forward—for the innovation in this field is one of detail.

John Horty
Chairman
Estes Park Institute

Preface

Hospitals and physicians are the infrastructure of the American health care system. What they do or don't do and how well or how poorly they do it directly affects every American. The problems and conflicts associated with the hospital-physician relationship are well known and well documented. Less well known and well documented are examples of successful relationships and the ingredients associated with their effectiveness. Our study's purpose was to identify some successful sites and uncover the reasons for their success. This book shares these reasons, lessons, guidelines, and best practices. The hope is that stronger partnerships can be built to deal with the challenges posed by American health care in the coming decade and beyond.

The approach taken was to probe beneath the surface for the underlying causes behind an effective relationship. What underlies what is observed? What is behind key events? Why is it that what works in one situation or setting does not work in another? What are the commonalities and differences? What are the root causes? It was a process similar to peeling an onion—stripping back layer upon layer of responses by repeatedly asking, why, what else, and what would be an example of that? The result, we hope, is a richness of experience that will be of interest and use to not only executives, physicians, and board members, but also policy makers and students of organizations.

To promote this objective, this book is written as an organizational semibiography. This approach emphasizes the participants telling their own story in their own words, making liberal use of direct quotes to illustrate relevant points and examples. Thus, the format of most chapters (particularly those in Part II and Part III) is to set the narrative stage by introducing the issues and providing overview comments, followed by the participants themselves sharing their experiences through their stories. The reader is encouraged to read these stories carefully, for herein "lies the gold." Attention should be paid to the words chosen, the ordering of words, the use of humor, and other nuances of language. These quotes should be read for their emotional tone as well as substantive content. Join with the participants as they share their struggles, their accomplishments, and their disappointments. For those, however, who cannot resist jumping ahead to the bottom line, or the punch line, most chapters contain concluding summaries of best practices, guidelines, and lessons that will help build more effective relationships. In addition, the introduction serves as an executive summary by highlighting the questions that formed the basis for the study and the key findings that resulted.

Part I (Defining the Relationship—Chapters 1 through 3) sets the stage by providing a historical context, outlining some conceptual models, and describing the study design. Part II (Managing the Relationship—Chapters 4 through 9) deals with fundamental issues of effectiveness, managerial style and decision-making approaches, communication, trust, conflict management, and change. Part III (Special Issues—Chapters 10 through 15) examines recurring challenges involving competition between hospitals and physicians, managed care, hospital-physician joint ventures, cost containment, nurse-physician relationships, and quality improvement Part IV (Building the Future—Chapters 16 and 17) describes several future issues likely to influence the relationship and what hospitals and physicians can do to better prepare for and influence their future.

We hope that readers will become users of the many ideas and guidelines shared by the ten sites and, in turn, will add to them. It is the behavior of hospitals and physicians that will come under increased public scrutiny in the coming years, and it is the behavior of hospitals and physicians in local communities that will largely determine the success or failure of the many quality improvement, cost containment, and access expansion policies currently under debate.

Acknowledgments

I am grateful to the Estes Park Institute and the Hospital Research and Educational Trust of the American Hospital Association for their support of this study. Appreciation is expressed to André Delbecq, Sandra Gill, and Spence Meighan of the Estes Park Institute and Linda Brooks and Monica Dreuth of the American Hospital Association for their assistance in conducting the site visit interviews and for providing many insights. Appreciation is also expressed to Donna Wilson of the American Hospital Association for her analysis of medical staff bylaws. Special recognition is due to the external advisory committee members: Dr. John Collins of Mercy Health Services; David Everhart, President Emeritus, Northwestern Memorial Hospital; Linda Haddad, Horty, Springer, and Mattern; John Horty, Chairman of the Board, Estes Park Institute; John Lowe, former Vice President, Hospital Research and Educational Trust, American Hospital Association; Charles Mason, Jr., President, Mills-Peninsula Hospital; Peter Schoenfeld, CEO, McPherson Community Health Center; and Dr. Richard YaDeau, Hospital Health Plan. The research assistance and staff support provided by Herb Buchanan, Tony Simons, Alice Schaller, and Cathy Ver Halen greatly facilitated analysis of the study data. I am also grateful for the supportive environment provided by the Graduate Program in Hospital and Health Services Management, J. L. Kellogg Graduate School of Management, and the Center for Health Services and Policy Research at Northwestern University.

The ultimate recognition, of course, is due the board members, executives, and physicians of the ten study sites who generously shared their time and experiences. I thank each of them by recognizing the CEOs who committed their institutions to the study: Mr. Robert Laverty, Catherine McAuley Health Center; Mr. James Mahar, Crouse-Irving Memorial Hospital; Ms. Jan Wyatt, Leonard Morse Hospital; Mr. Ken Schull, Lexington Medical Center; Mr. Arlen Reynolds, North Monroe Hospital; Mr. Peter Bigelow, Providence Medical Center; Mr. Ames Early and Mr. Martin Buser, Scripps Memorial Hospital; Mr. Patrick Hays, Sutter Health; Mr. Donald Shropshire, Tucson Medical Center; and Mr. Ron LaBott, West Allis Memorial Hospital.

Portions of this study—Chapters 6, 7, 8, and 9 concerning communication, trust, managing conflicts, and managing change—were prepared as a part of a Fellowship Project for the American College of Healthcare Executives.

Introduction

The idea for the study began with a number of questions that were being asked with increasing frequency regarding the current state of hospital-physician relationships. These questions and their responses are used as the format for summarizing some of the study's key findings. Each question is cross-referenced to a specific chapter where the reader will find an extended discussion of the issue along with many examples, illustrations, lessons, and guidelines.

1. What are some of the main themes or messages associated with developing more effective hospital-physician relationships? (See Chapter 17.)

The most pervasive theme of the study was the importance of a culture that emphasizes working jointly with physicians in pursuing the institution's mission and objectives. This was reflected in early and ongoing physician involvement in strategic planning and implementation; a genuine respect for and liking of physicians; open, honest, and persistent communication; investment in developing strong physician leadership, including grooming younger physicians to assume future leadership roles; a willingness to explore alternative organizational forms; an ability to work together as business partners; and a knack for managing the pace of change. Various chapters throughout the book contain examples of specific approaches associated with the above themes.

I am grateful to André Delbecq for suggesting the question and answer format as a way of summarizing the study results.

2. What constitutes an effective relationship? What criteria are used? (See Chapter 4.)

Respondents tended to use two general sets of criteria for defining an effective relationship: process criteria and outcome criteria. Among the most salient process criteria were frequent, honest, and open communication; the ability to tackle tough issues together; and the ability to move on things—to address problems in a timely fashion. Among the most important outcome criteria mentioned were the ability to develop successful joint ventures; the ability to maintain and increase patient volume and market share; and the ability to maintain standards of clinical accountability.

3. What are some of the more effective ways of involving physicians in management and governance? How does one groom younger physicians to assume leadership roles? (See Chapter 5.)

A comprehensive approach of involving physicians in management and governance activities throughout the organization appears to be most successful. At the heart of this is the early and ongoing involvement of physicians in the strategic planning process of the institution. Creation of a full-time medical director/executive vice president for medical affairs position is helpful. In addition to the usual quality assurance responsibilities, individuals filling these positions can play a key role in implementing strategies of joint interest to the hospital and physicians. The sites also found retreats to be a particularly effective mechanism of physician involvement. Most sites found it increasingly important to reimburse physicians for taking on expanded managerial responsibilities.

A key aspect of grooming younger physicians to assume future leadership roles is to show them that the hospital really cares about their professional success. This means identifying their career interests and moving to meet them with a variety of practice assistance and enhancement programs. In this way, younger physicians begin to recognize the interdependence between themselves and the hospital in a way that is meaningful to them. It then becomes easier to involve them in hospital committee work, in the activities of parallel organizations such as independent practice associations and joint physician-hospital organizations, and in eventually assuming larger leadership responsibility. A number of specific mechanisms can be used, ranging from the assignment of administrators to work with selected younger physicians (a "buddy system") to the creation of nonvoting positions on the medical staff executive committee so that younger physicians can learn more about the larger issues facing the hospital and its medical staff.

4. What are some of the more effective approaches for facilitating communication between hospitals and physicians? (See Chapter 6.)

Effective communication is based in large part on understanding how
others learn and process information—spending time with people in
order to get to know them. Both rich (face-to-face) and lean (the written
word) forms of communication are important. Factual information helps
to reduce uncertainty, while face-to-face discussion helps to deal with
complex and ambiguous issues.

It is also important to communicate the larger context of a message
or decision, for example, why a decision such as developing a physician
office building may be delayed and what contingencies may need to be
anticipated.

Among some of the approaches used to enhance communication
were the development of communication protocols (such as returning
physician telephone calls promptly); anticipating bad news in order to
eliminate surprises; and particpating in communication training
workshops.

5. What are the most important ingredients for developing a trusting
   relationship? (See Chapter 7.)

Trust is developed through both shared values and meeting each other's
legitimate self-interests. It is developed by open, honest communication; following through on what one says one is going to do; and providing a sense of fairness. It is also assisted by a stable top-management
team; the presence of a medical director and strong physician leadership; and the recognition that trust is fragile. It must be reearned on a
daily basis using every opportunity presented.

6. What are some of the more effective ways of managing conflict? (See
   Chapter 8.)

For the most part, open, collaborative problem-solving approaches
proved to be most effective for dealing with conflict issues. Such an
approach was characterized by focusing on the problem rather than
personalities, clarifying roles and expectations, providing full information, and seeking the best solution to the problem given the circumstances. What did not work was trying to move too fast on a given issue,
not involving the right people, placing too much responsibility on a few
physician leaders, failing to address a problem at the appropriate level in
the organization, and not directly confronting issues.

7. How did the study sites manage change? (See Chapter 9.)

The most effective efforts at managing change recognized the need to align hospital and physician strategies with various structures and day-to-day decision-making processes in order to deal with environmental forces. This meant defining the current state of affairs, assessing the degree of discomfort with the current state, articulating the future desired state that a sufficient number of people could accept, and then developing the implementation plans and ongoing support mechanisms to bring about the change. It was particularly important to manage the pace of change—that is, when to speed it up as well as when to slow it down.

8. How was the issue of competition between hospitals and physicians handled? (See Chapter 10.)

Among the approaches that the study sites found most helpful in dealing with hospital-physician competition were

1. advance planning and consultation (often through the strategic planning process) with a strong role played by medical staff leadership
2. using parallel organizations, such as independent practice associations (IPAs) and physician-hospital organizations (PHOs) to discuss potentially competitive issues
3. using the threat of the outside environment (the common-enemy approach) to encourage cooperative rather than competitive behavior
4. not overreacting to physician competitive threats against the hospital

Hospitals recognized the long-run implications of the relationship and, where possible, attempted to head off physician competition through developing joint ventures.

9. How did the sites handle the challenges posed by managed care? (See Chapter 11.)

Issues involving managed care were among the most frequently reported challenges by study respondents. Among the more effective approaches were those that recognized the importance of developing business partnerships that could present a united front to outside purchasers. Strong physician-led cost containment/utilization review practices were also essential. Other successul ingredients included using an organizational mechanism, such as an IPA or PHO, to sort through and negotiate managed care options; recognizing that managed care is a business; and demonstrating the need for a strong primary care physician base.

10. What were the sites' experiences in regard to hospital-physician joint ventures? (See Chapter 12.)

At least eight of the sites became involved in hospital-physician economic joint ventures. The more successful were those in which

1. both hospitals and physicians were at financial risk
2. the joint venture provided a strategic fit with both hospital and physician plans
3. explicit review criteria were developed that included a detailed business plan with specific contingencies spelled out in the event that performance did not meet expectations
4. investment opportunities were made available to all interested physicians (exclusivity was avoided) as well as to outside investors (to dilute physician ownership interests)
5. the joint venture was managed as a professional business relationship

11. What were the sites' experiences in regard to cost containment? (See Chapter 13.)

While all sites were involved in cost-containment activities, they were not a major source of hospital-physician conflict. As much, if not more, emphasis was given to working with physicians to create additional revenue and market share opportunities. Effective cost-containment practices were those that

1. had substantial physician involvement
2. emphasized the link between cost-effective use of resources and quality of care
3. linked utilization review activities with risk management and quality assurance activities
4. made staff cuts in areas not directly affecting patient care
5. provided ongoing education regarding the need for cost-effective patient care

12. Given the changes occurring in both professions, what was the status of relationships between physicians and nurses? (See Chapter 14.)

Perhaps the most surprising finding of the study was the extent of conflict between physicians and nurses. Almost all of the sites noted physician-nurse conflict as a problem requiring considerable attention. Many had appointed special nurse-physician liaison committees or task forces to deal with the issues. Other approaches included targeting selected physicians to act as mediators with problem physicians, developing a nursing futures task force, establishing communication protocols, and using focus groups drawing on the assistance of outside facilitators.

13. Given the new demands for clinical accountability, what are the sites doing in the area of quality assurance, assessment, and improvement? (See Chapter 15.)

All sites had moved to strengthen their credentialing process. Some developed joint board–medical staff policy review committees composed of both board members and physicians. Half of the sites used computerized physician performance profile data in considering physicians for renewal of privileges. The remaining sites were planning to do so. All sites were upgrading their quality assurance processes and giving greater attention to integrating quality assurance with risk management and utilization review. In addition, considerable effort was given to integrating hospitalwide quality assurance efforts with medical staff quality assurance activities. A couple of the sites were involved in continuous quality improvement programs.

14. What do the sites see as the main challenges facing the hospital-physician relationship in the future? (See Chapter 16.)

Respondents generally felt that the next few years would be even more challenging than the past. In addition to the continued emphasis on containing costs, respondents noted the new challenge of maintaining and improving quality. For most, being able to survive (and thrive) in a managed care world posed a major challenge. They also saw challenges in trying to create effective joint ventures with their physicians, developing new organizational forms to deal with the continually changing environment, recruiting additional primary care physicians, and developing various physician practice assistance programs to help better position physicians to meet the changing environmental demands.

PART I

Defining the Relationship

CHAPTER 1

Contextual Factors Affecting Hospital-Physician Relationships

> The relationship between the hospital and medical staff will become increasingly difficult as competitive pressures build and as managed care becomes increasingly prevalent. Resolution of these issues will depend on hospital CEOs demonstrating strong leadership in aligning the interest of their institution with those of payers, insurers, patients, and physicians. In many instances, the interests of these groups are so varied that conflict inevitably will result. However, strong hospital/physician relations will likely be a critical factor in determining whether hospitals survive the next five years of structural change and intense competition. (Amara, Morrison, and Schmid 1988).

Hospital-physician relationships have long been influenced by economic, social, political, and cultural factors. This chapter provides a historical context for examining the influence of these factors on the relationship between hospitals and physicians.

The destinies of hospitals and physicians are intertwined in complex and paradoxical ways. At the center of the paradox is the fact that more of the relationship will be defined by what occurs *outside* of the traditionally defined hospital. What it means to be a hospital and what it means to practice medicine are being reinvented in response to new economic, technological, and societal forces. (Eisele, Fifer, and Wilson 1985). Among the pressures most intensely felt by the ten sites studied were

1. the inadequacy of Medicare reimbursement
2. general cost containment and reimbursement pressures from employers and third party payers
3. dealing with HMOs and related managed care contracting

4. malpractice costs

5. regulatory pressures

6. the increased competition for patients on the part of both hospitals and physicians

The success of hospitals and physicians in dealing with these and related pressures will be largely determined by their ability to

1. understand the context (that is, the environmental forces) within which they are operating

2. understand each other's cultures, values, and goals

3. develop partnership-building skills including communication, trust, managing conflict, and coping with change

THE HISTORICAL CONTEXT

The current state of hospital-physician relationships is not simply the product of recent changes in health care policies. Rather, it has been shaped by decades of events and experiences going back to the turn of the century. At least six of the ten sites had a number of key third-generation physicians in their late 50s and early 60s. These physicians began practicing in the late 1960s and at that time were strongly influenced by a second generation of physicians trained in the 1930s and the 1940s, who, in turn, were products of exposure to first-generation physicians, who trained and practiced in the early 1900s. Even physicians associated with the hospitals founded in more recent times are products of exposure to physicians and a medical culture of earlier time periods, as experienced through the historical traces present in graduate medical education and postgraduate residency programs. The historical traces may be categorized into four time periods as shown in Table 1.1. The time periods are approximate only and are not meant to imply abrupt or clean breaks from one time period to another.

Physician-Owned (1900–1930)

Since there was relatively little that could be done to treat patients, hospitals in the early 1900s were largely custodial in nature. Since such care took relatively little time, physicians, their nurses, or both could oversee hospital operations. Many hospitals were, in fact, owned by physicians, particularly in smaller communities and suburbs. In some cases, physicians started their own hospitals in response to being shut out of other hospitals in the area that utilized closed staffs (Starr 1982,

Table 1.1 The Historical Context of Hospital-Physician Relationships

	1900–1929	1930–1973	1974–1985	1986–Future
Government role	Essentially none	Expansion of coverage for the elderly, medically indigent, and special categorical groups	Increased regulation of hospital operating costs and capital expenditures — for example, the 1974 Health Planning and Resource Development Act, the 1983 Medicare Prospective Payment legislation	Further governmental expansion into regulation of costs and quality of care
Hospital payment	Private paid patients, charity, and philanthropy	Third-party commercial insurance and government reimbursement	Growing reimbursement from federal and state government under fixed prices and under managed care contract from private insurers	Continued growth in fixed prices and discounting; continued pressure to contain costs
Physician payment	Private pay patients	Third-party commercial insurance and government reimbursement	Continued payment based on prevailing reasonable and customary charges	Move toward payment based on relative value scales and expenditure caps on physician services component

Continued

Table 1.1 Continued

	1900–1929	1930–1973	1974–1985	1986–Future
Technology	Minimal; essentially pretechnology era	Breakthroughs in asepsis techniques lead to marked increase in surgery and hospital utilization, followed by subsequent rapid advances in drugs and related therapies for patient treatment	Continued rapid technological growth particularly in invasive procedures and surgical techniques, bioengineering, etc.	Rapid growth in technology permitting more outpatient treatment; less invasive surgery; monoclonal antibodies, lasers, etc.
Site of patient treatment	Largely at home and physician's office	Largely based in physician's office and the hospital	In hospitals, single specialty and multispecialty group practices and clinics, nursing homes and aftercare facilities	Physician groups and clinics, patient's home, work settings, aftercare sites, and hospitals
Nature of hospital-physician relationship	Physician owned and/or managed hospitals	Physicians control hospital through patient admission and medical staff organization	Managers exert greater control over resources affecting how physicians practice medicine; regulations begin to create competing incentives for hospitals and physicians	Search for more joint control, mutual influence, and shared authority in order to cope with increasingly complex demands; search for a new form of health care organization

157). The arrangement worked well, since payment, for the most part, came directly from patients with no intermediaries involved in the process. Since the center of medical care during this period was largely the patient's home or the physician's office, the hospital (with the exception of the developing teaching hospitals) played a relatively minor role, and opportunities for conflict between hospitals and physicians were essentially nonexistent.

Physician-Controlled (1930–1974)

As advances in diagnosis and treatment emerged, coupled with the growth of governmental financed care and private health insurance coverage, physicians found themselves with more patients and an ability to do more for these patients. Practicing medicine became a busier activity. Many physicians found themselves no longer able to both run a busy practice and oversee an increasingly complex set of hospital activities. As a result, they turned over many of the administrative activities to nonclinically trained administrators or superintendents while maintaining control by organizing themselves as "medical staffs" with defined rights and privileges as well as responsibilities. It is important to note that the real power of the formally organized medical staff was in the ability of its individual members to admit patients. The goal of the hospital administrators and superintendents was, indeed, to keep the medical staff satisfied by running a smoothly operating workshop for its practitioners. During this period, physicians did not need to own the hospital since they could effectively control it through their ability to influence hospital admissions and through their political power, represented by the medical staff organization. Further, most community hospitals, eager for patients during this period, opened up the opportunity for privileges to any qualified physician, thus removing the incentive for physicians to own their own hospital (Starr 1982, 218, 219). This was also a relatively stable period in which the external forces were largely supportive of such a relationship. The hospital was reimbursed its charges, the hospital was a primary target for local community philanthropy, and what little regulation existed did not pit hospital and physician against each other.

Even the introduction of Medicare in 1965, which was fought by the American Medical Association and many individual physicians, did not upset the fundamental physician control of the hospital-physician relationship. In fact, both hospitals and physicians benefited financially by receiving reimbursement for patients who previously could not pay for their care. And while the Darling decision (1965), establishing the hospital's board of trustees as ultimately responsible for the quality of care, upgraded the power and authority of hospital boards, few knew how to appropriately act on this authority. Thus, most medical staffs were left free to conduct business as usual.

Manager-Controlled (1974–1985)

The sentinel event signaling a fundamental change in the nature of the hospital-physician relationship was the passage of the Health Planning and Development Act of 1974. This act established local and state health systems agencies charged with the responsibility for approving capital expenditures for new services and programs beyond defined dollar limits. For the first time, decisions regarding new technologies and expansion of facilities were subjected to external review. Hospitals expanded their administrative planning staffs—a move viewed by many physicians as a grab for more power and control. Physicians began to lose some control over important decisions affecting their livelihood and their relationship with the hospital. Administrators began to move to center stage, playing a more pivotal role in the allocation of medical resources. When requests were turned down or scaled down, administrators became a visible and unwilling target for physician wrath.

At the same time, many states initiated rate review programs designed to control increases in hospital operating costs. In these states hospitals felt pressures to manage more efficiently, which placed administrators and physicians at cross purposes. Rate review programs gave more power, authority, and control to management, while physicians continued to lose control.

The final major development during this period was, of course, the passage of Medicare Prospective Payment in 1983. While limited to Medicare patients, for the first time all hospitals had to respond to systemic incentives to contain costs and to solicit physician cooperation in this endeavor. In contrast, physicians had no such incentive. Concurrent with the introduction of Medicare Prospective Payment were the continued growth of new technologies permitting more patients to be treated on an outpatient basis, the growth of health maintenance organizations and managed care plans, pressures from employers to contain costs, and an increase in the supply of physicians. The net result was that physicians were not only continuing to lose control over what went on in the hospital (Perrow 1963) but were also faced with pressures to modify how they practiced medicine in their offices. This sense of loss involved not only a diminished ability to control and shape their professional destiny and, therefore, economic well-being but also represented a blow to their sense of craftsmanship and ability to utilize their skills to the fullest, as reflected in the following physician's comments (Sheldon 1986, 55):

> The particular role of the physician is as much art as science. Being in a position to understand people who are ill from the perspective of the biological, psychological, and sociological. So far a well-trained physician remains the person in our society capable of helping in those three dimensions simultaneously, and if anything is done to make physicians mere biomedical technicians while the psycho-social side of medical care is taken over by social workers or nurse practitioners that will be a net loss for patients.
>
> It is being a person, a human, not a machine or a computer that spits out medicine and diagnoses. Anything that is going to change the doctor-patient relationship in terms of my ability to deal with them on a one-to-one basis is going to upset me. And anything that takes away my right to handle or deal with patients and their problems in a personal manner is going to upset me. If I have to do it from an administrator's standpoint or cost-effective standpoint rather than what I think is best for them, then I am going to be upset. Those are ideals of medicine for me.

Or as expressed by one study physician:

> I love sick people. I love human nature and enjoy being worthy. The patient has no advocate unless the advocate is his doctor. The nurse cares, the lab technician cares, the administrator cares, but when it comes down to push and shove, the physician must sit up on his hind legs and growl until he gets what he needs to take care of his sick patient.

In forging ahead to meet the challenges of the new environment, hospital executives and policymakers should not ignore or underestimate the multiple sense of loss that many physicians are experiencing (Gill 1989). As one study physician exclaimed: "Physicians are so paranoid now as you know from talking to me. Oh my God, this is a group of people for whom everything seems out of control. It is so real and growing everyday . . . anything that happens right now is a real threat."

Joint Control (1985–Future)

Most hospital executives recognize the folly of attempting to position their organization to meet the challenges of the new environment without significant physician involvement. As a result, a new period of hospital-physician relationships is beginning to emerge that has been variously described as conjoint (Scott 1982) or shared authority (Shortell 1983, 1985). It is characterized by greater physician involvement in the governance and management of the institution, including determination of the hospital's strategic plan and objectives and the allocation of resources to meet those objectives. It is reinforced by the new Joint Commission on Accreditation of Healthcare Organizations' principles of organizational effectiveness, emphasizing integrated board, administrative, and clinical leadership of the institution at all levels.

For example, in the ten sites studied, nine involve physicians as voting members of the hospital's governing board, and all ten have moderate to extensive physician involvement in the strategic planning process. Five sites had salaried or part-time medical directors or executive vice presidents for medical affairs, three had full-time or part-time paid section chiefs, three had physicians occupying other salaried administrative positions in the hospital (for example, vice president for strategic planning), six had economic joint venture relationships with their physicians, seven had parallel organization structures such as a joint physician-hospital organization, and eight had at least two-year terms of offices for the president of the staff to insure greater continuity of involvement and leadership.

While extensive, these efforts were met with varying degrees of success. One major reason was that the definition of, and expectations for, involvement on the part of the hospital board and management were sometimes quite different from the definition of, and expectations for, involvement on the part of physicians. For example, the board and management may desire physician input on such strategies as expanding the primary care base in terms of refining the idea and helping to make it work. Some physicians, in contrast, desire *early* involvement in the process, including discussion of the underlying assumptions about the need for the program in the first place. What the board and management views as "involvement" is often perceived by some physicians as "token participation."

A second issue facing hospitals and physicians is the difficulty that the medical staff leadership faces in attempting to speak for the majority of active physicians on the staff. While many of the study sites developed creative ways of communicating with the staff physicians in attempting to represent their viewpoints, all acknowledged that it was a challenging task. Often as many as 15 to 20 physician leaders would be involved early and continually in the decision-making process, but there appeared to be little carryover effect to the majority of physicians on the staff. It somehow did not permeate the organization or trickle down. In some cases, the staff were not even aware of the degree of involvement on the part of the staff leadership. In other cases, the awareness did not seem to translate into anything that was seen as meaningful to the individual physician's needs or professional career. This gap between physician leadership involvement and staff apathy or, in some cases, alienation was present in most sites. In one site, it became a major issue: The medical staff at large, dissatisfied with the current medical staff executive committee leadership, voted to establish a new organization to represent their interests, thereby replacing the existing leadership. While the proposal did not pass, the closeness of the vote indicated the prevalence and strength of the concern.

A third major challenge to the joint control model is the reeognition that physicians and managers are socialized and trained differently, resulting in different world views and value orientations. The following section contrasts these along important dimensions involving the basis of knowledge, orientation toward time, orientation toward patients, rules of evidence, and related criteria. The growth of hospital systems and the corporate office-hospital relationship adds an additional level of complexity to the individual hospital-physician relationship.

A fourth challenge, of course, involves the many external pressures facing both hospitals and physicians. As resources become more scarce, as payment programs tighten, and as managed care programs grow, hospitals and physicians increasingly see themselves as competing for their share of a common smaller pie. For example, in a recent study of 600 hospital executives, 62 percent reported that competition for outpatients was the leading cause of hospital-physician conflict, with managed care activities also a significant source (Grayson and McCormick 1988). At least two of the study hospitals found themselves in serious conflict with a significant number of physicians over reimbursement issues involving HMOs. The physicians felt that their reimbursement and collections relative to the hospital portion were too low.

Given the implementation of physician payment schedules based on relative values and the likelihood of expenditure targets, the economic pressures on physicians will increase significantly in coming years. Issues of income inequality by specialty are likely to lead to increased conflict among physicians themselves. In addition, growing concerns over the ethical issues of physician ownership involvement in institutions to which they make referrals (U.S. Congress 1989) are likely to place increased stress on the hospital-physician relationship as both groups seek new ways of forging economic partnerships. These factors will lead to increased physician activity to expand their revenue base and lower their costs—behavior that will offer both opportunities and challenges to hospitals. Those discussions will primarily involve out-of-hospital care, and it is in this area that the joint control approach will be tested. No longer is the issue who will control the hospital, but rather who will control the delivery system from the patient's home to the physician's office, to the hospital, to the postacute facility, and back again to the patient's home. The increase in the volume of outpatient activity is well documented by a recent study showing that while in 1983 about two-thirds of Medicare physician dollars were spent in the hospital, in 1986 it had fallen to under one-half (Mitchell, Wedig, and Cromwell 1989). In the same study, the percentage of spending in the physician's office rose from 29 to 33 percent, while the share spent in outpatient departments and ambulatory surgical centers almost tripled from 6 to 15 percent. By 1986, Medicare beneficiaries were spending nearly 30 percent more for physicians' services than in 1983.

In summary, the emerging model of joint control will be strongly tested. Personal values, economic pressures, competitive uncertainty, and difficulties in hospital-physician communication all pose serious challenges to conjoint leadership.

THE CULTURAL CONTEXT

There are two important cultural distinctions to be made. The first involves the cultural differences between managers and physicians. The second involves the differences between corporate management and the individual entrepreneur. Each is highlighted below.

Table 1.2 summarizes some of the primary cultural distinctions between managers and physicians. These differences have their roots in both the self-selection of individuals into different careers and the different training and socialization experiences associated with professional education itself (Kurtz 1987). For health care executives, the underlying basis of knowledge is primarily the social and management sciences (economics, sociology, quantitative methods, finance, marketing, organization behavior, etc.), while for physicians the primary basis is the biomedical sciences. The patient focus of executives is typically broad, encompassing all patients in the organization today as well as the larger community from which future patients may be derived. In contrast, the physicians' focus is much narrower: The concern is with individual patients and their immediate needs. In regard to exposure to other health professionals and patients while in training, health care executives typically receive relatively little exposure, while physicians receive a great deal. In contrast, physicians receive almost no exposure in training to the larger business/economic world of health care. The time frame of action for the health care executive is typically longer than for physicians. The executives' strategic responsibility to position the organization vis-à-vis the environment requires a long-run focus and orientation (while still attending to daily operations); physicians are much more short-run oriented—in part, due to the need to solve immediate clinical problems facing their patients. The two groups also have different views of "evidence." While both managerial decision making and clinical decision making are fraught with ambiguity and uncertainty, the training and background of the health care executive leads to a greater acceptance of "soft" qualitative data and loosely linked cause-and-effect relationships upon which to base decisions, while the training and

Table 1.2 Cultural Differences between Health Care Executives and Physicians

Attribute	Health Care Executives	Physicians
Basis of knowledge	Primarily social and management sciences	Primarily biomedical sciences
Exposure to relevant others while in training	Relatively little exposure to physicians, nurses, other heath care professionals, or patients	Great deal of exposure to nurses, other health care professionals, and patients; little exposure to broader business/economic world of health care
Patient focus	Broad: all patients in the organization and the larger community	Narrow: one's individual patients
Time frame of action	Middle to long run; emphasis on positioning the organization for the future	Generally short run; meet immediate needs of patients
Rules of evidence	Understand the need to act on "soft" qualitative information; loose-linked cause–effect relationships that may not be well understood	"Soft" qualitative information viewed with skepticism; prefer "hard" facts; tightly linked cause–effect relationships that are well understood
View of resources	Always limited; challenge lies in allocating scarce resources efficiently and effectively	Resources essentially unlimited or at least should be unlimited; resources should be availble to maximize the quality of care
Professional identity	Less cohesive; less well developed	More cohesive; highly developed

background of the physician leads to suspicion of such rationales and a preference for "hard" scientific facts with tight cause-and-effect relationships. The two groups also differ in their view of resources: Administrators view them as always limited, with every decision always involving trade-offs and opportunity costs, while many physicians still view resources as essentially unlimited, particularly when it comes to doing everything they can for their own patients. Finally, the two groups differ in the extent to which they identify with their professions. Health care executives typically have a much less cohesive sense of professional identity relative to the highly developed sense of professional identity of physicians.

The above distinctions may be somewhat overdrawn, and there are, of course, exceptions as well as differences by both medical specialty and type of health care executive. Surgeons, for example, tend to have a narrower patient focus and shorter time frame of action than most internists or family practitioners (Sheldon 1986, 203–204). On the administrative side, chief operating officers and middle managers are likely to have a shorter time frame of action and narrower view of hospital activities than will the president or chief executive officer. Other differences will exist in terms of line versus staff responsibilities. Nonetheless, the distinctions drawn are generally on target, are pervasive, and have extremely important implications for the hospital-physician relationship. The world of management and the world of medicine contain different "tribes," each with its own language, values, culture, thought patterns, and rules of the game (Neuhauser 1988). It is important for both managers and physicians to recognize and work with these differences. Each comes from a different background and professional socialization experience. Each has a different time frame of action, ways of viewing evidence, concept of what is persuasive, and a different view of resources and how they might be used. Each has a different view of patients, of the larger community, and a somewhat different sense of professional identity. Neither is inherently right or wrong, nor is one orientation better than the other. But they are different. One of the lessons of this book is that these differences, if recognized and worked with, can become a key strength of the relationship. The demanding health care environment of the future requires a diversity of orientations, approaches, skills, and experiences to be successful. The key lies in working with the differences. Examples and guidelines for doing this are discussed in Part II.

In addition to the above basic cultural differences between managers and physicians, there are also differences that have been created by the rise of the health care corporation, reflected primarily in the growth of hospital systems (Shortell 1988). As a result, the individual hospital-physician relationship is now embedded within the context of a larger relationship between the corporate office (sometimes regional or divisional offices) and individual hospital members. This gives rise to additional opportunities for conflict and misunderstanding between the wishes of the corporate office attempting to represent systemwide interests and the goals and objectives of individual hospitals and their associated physician members (Shalowitz and Shortell 1988). As discussed in subsequent chapters, this is particularly true in regard to individual hospital-physician joint venture opportunities, HMO development, and managed care contracts, where the interests and desires of local hospitals and physician entrepreneurs can run counter to the systemwide plans of the corporate office. Some systems have attempted to bridge this gap and deal with these issues by developing corporatewide offices or divisions of physician affairs directed by physicians and charged with the responsibility of integrating and aligning local hospital-physician initiatives and those of the system (Shortell, Morrison, and Friedman 1990).

CURRENT STATUS OF THE RELATIONSHIP

It is widely acknowledged that hospital-physician relationships are in a state of flux (Grayson 1988). Some observers infer from this that the relationship has seriously deteriorated and may be incapable of dealing with the many challenges facing the field. Clearly, the effectiveness of the traditional medical staff organization to deal with the newly emerging economic forces has been seriously questioned (Fifer 1987; Shortell 1983, 1985).

Yet, despite these concerns, recent studies strike a ray of hope. For example, Georgopoulos, D'Aunno, and Saavedra (1987) found hospital-physician relationships to remain good after introduction of a prepayment program that posed great challenges to the relationship. In a national survey of several hundred hospitals, the Joint Commission on Accreditation of Healthcare Organizations (JCAHO) found that 79 percent of hospitals reported significant disagreement over the period 1985–1987, but more than 80 percent were satisfied with the relationship (JCAHO 1988). In fact, over 60 percent felt the relationship had been improving over the two-year period, with an even higher percentage believing the relationship would continue to improve over the coming five years. These findings were essentially confirmed by a 1987 Hamilton/KSA study of 753 CEOs, in which 54 percent believed their relationship with medical staff members had improved (Grayson 1988). In the Joint Commission study, the most frequently reported unresolved differences related to (1) physician recruitment, (2) malpractice insurance, (3) availability of specific services, and (4) acquisition of new technology. Adverse financial pressures were reported as having the most negative impact on the relationship, while four factors were most favorably cited as having a positive impact: (1) having each group fulfill its responsibilities, (2) good communication, (3) sensitivity in relationships, and (4) mutual involvement in decision making.

Based on the present study, there appear to be two primary reasons for the disparity between public perceptions of hospital-physician relationships and the recent data. The first is the tendency to confuse problems or conflict as evidence of a poor relationship. There is a tendency among health care organizations, and particularly board members, to equate an effective organization with the absence of conflict or problems. This is, in part, due to the more tranquil environment of the 1950s and 1960s, when the roles and responsibilities of the board, management, and medical staff were more clearly drawn, and the hospital could essentially achieve its objectives by keeping physicians happy. But, in today's turbulent health care environment, problems and conflict are inevitable and do not, in and of themselves, signal a poor or deteriorating relationship. Rather, the strength of the relationship lies in whether or not the problems are surfaced and the conflicts dealt with openly. The success of the relationship is determined by the ability to address the most important problems and manage conflict effectively so that these problems do not linger, and hospitals and physicians are able to move forward in achieving their objectives. Thus, in the Joint Commission's survey, while over 80 percent indicated they were satisfied with the relationship, 79 percent reported that they, indeed, faced significant problems. In present times, the absence of problems and conflict would be suspect, indicating an organization refusing to acknowledge its problems. As will become evident in later chapters, how hospitals and physicians dealt with their problems and conflicts (see Part II and Part III) was a key indicator of an effective relationship, not the absence of problems and conflict.

A second reason for the disparity between public perception and recent data involves the transition that many hospitals and physicians are making in their relationship as they cope with changes in the environment. These changes, which are examined throughout this book, cause problems and conflict but, at the same time, provide mechanisms, opportunities, and forums for discussion, debate, and involvement toward resolving conflict and searching for common ground. Thus, respondents in both surveys felt that, if anything, relationships were getting stronger and would likely be even better in the near future, although not without being sorely tested. This conclusion is generally supported by the present findings reported in this book.

Given the current health care environment, the hospital-physician relationship can probably best be described as one of high risk and high reward. While the federal government and other third party payers are playing an increasingly dominant role in the development of health policy, it must be remembered that hospitals and physicians are the primary instruments through which those policies are implemented. The ability of the U.S. health care system to adapt to the changing demands will be largely determined by how well hospitals and physicians work together. A recent study of 162 CEOs revealed that the lack of physician commitment was the most frequent reason given for the failure of hospital projects, and ineffective administrator-physician relationships were also cited as a leading factor (second only to reimbursement constraints) contributing to industrywide hospital failures (Boyle 1988). Physicians are beginning to experience similar consequences. The stakes are indeed high. What is required is a redefinition of the hospital-physician relationship along multiple lines—clinical, economic, ethical, legal, and organizational. This will require a new form of social contract based on mutual involvement and shared authority and influence. Some models of newly emerging relationships are discussed further in the next chapter.

REFERENCES

Amara, R., J. J. Morrison, and G. Schmid. 1988. *Looking Ahead at American Health Care*. Washington, DC: McGraw-Hill.

Boyle, R. L. 1988. "Will You Be Singing in the Rain?" *Health Care Forum Journal* (September/October):10–18.

Darling, V. 1965. Charleston Community Memorial Hospital, 211 N.E. Second 253.

Eisele, C. W., W. R. Fifer, and T. C. Wilson. 1985. *The Medical Staff and the Modern Hospital*. Englewood, CO: Estes Park Institute.

Fifer, W. R. 1987. "The Hospital Medical Staff of 1997," *Quality Review Bulletin* (June):194–97.

Georgopoulos, B. S., T. A. D'Aunno, and R. Saavedra. 1987. "Hospital-Physician Relations under Hospital Prepayment," *Medical Care* 25(August):781–95.

Gill, S. L. 1989. "The Physician Executive and Professional Grief," *Physician Executive* (March-April):8–17.

Grayson, M. A. 1988. "Survey Spots the Tight Turns in M.D.-CEO Relations," *Hospitals* (February 5):48–53.

Grayson, M. A., and B. McCormick. 1988. "Outpatients a Source of M.D./Hospital Conflict," *Medical Staff Leader* 18(March):1.

Joint Commission on Accreditation of Healthcare Organizations. 1988. *Report of the Joint Commission Survey of Relationships among Governing Bodies, Management, and Medical Staffs in U.S. Hospitals*. Chicago, IL: JCAHO.

Kurtz, M. E. 1987. "Role of the Physician as Manager," *Physical Medicine and Rehabilitation: State of the Art Reviews* 1, 2:185–96.

Mitchell, J., G. Wedig, and J. Cromwell. 1989. "The Medicare Physician Fee Freeze: What Really Happened?" *Health Affairs* 8:21–33.

Neuhauser, P. C. 1988. *Tribal Warfare in Organizations.* Cambridge, MA: Ballinger Publishing.

Perrow, C. 1963. "Goals and Power Structure: A Historical Case Study," in E. Freidson (Ed.), *The Hospital in Modern Society.* Glencoe, IL: Free Press.

Scott, W. R. 1982. "Managing Professional Work: Three Models of Control for Health Organizations," *Health Services Research* 17:213–40.

Shalowitz, J. I., and S. M. Shortell. 1988. "The Emerging Roles of Physicians in Health Care Systems," Chicago, IL: American Hospital Association, Health Systems Division, 29–54.

Sheldon, A. 1986. *Managing Doctors.* Homewood, IL: Dow Jones–Irwin.

Shortell, S. M. 1983. "Physician Involvement in Hospital Decision-Making," in B. Gray (Ed.), *The New Health Care For Profit.* Washington, DC: The National Academy Press, Institute of Medicine, 73–102.

———. 1985. "The Medical Staff of the Future: Replanting the Garden," *Frontiers of Health Services Management* 1(February):3–48. Also reprinted in A. R. Kovner and D. Neuhauser (Eds.), *Health Services Management: Readings and Commentary.* 3rd ed. Ann Arbor, MI: Health Administration Press, 1987, 248–76.

———. 1988. "The Evolution of Hospital Systems: Unfulfilled Promises and Self-Fulfilling Prophecies," *Medical Care Review* 45(2):177–214.

Shortell, S. M., E. M. Morrison, and B. Friedman. 1990. *Strategic Choices for America's Hospitals: Managing Change in Turbulent Times.* San Francisco: Jossey-Bass.

Starr, P. 1982. *The Social Transformation of American Medicine.* New York: Basic Books.

U.S. Congress. 1989. *Ethics in Patient Referral Act of 1989.* H.R. 939.

CHAPTER 2

Models of the Hospital-Physician Relationship

Much of the ambiguity and paradox in the hospital-physician relationship is due to the fact that most physicians are not hospital employees, and yet they exert dominant control over the use of hospital resources. Two major perspectives—derived from economics and organization theory—help to shed light on this fact and set the stage for a better understanding of the experiences, guidelines, and lessons discussed in Part II and Part III.

Economists have typically viewed the relationship in terms of the physician as buyer and the hospital as seller of services (Newhouse 1970; Pauly and Redisch 1973; Pauly 1980; Harris 1977). The relationship can also be viewed from the perspective of principal and agent (Fama and Jensen 1986). Physicians can serve as the hospital's agent, as in the case of providing emergency room coverage; conversely, the hospital can serve as the physician's agent, as in the case of purchasing new medical technology. Organization theorists have typically viewed the relationship as a loosely coupled professional bureaucracy (Smith 1955: Mintzberg 1979; Scott 1982; Shortell 1985). Whether economic-based or organization theory–based, a key concept governing the relationship is the notion of *transaction costs* (Williamson 1975, 1985). Transaction costs are those costs incurred by hospitals and physicians in the process of working together. They include the time spent by physicians in committee work and quality assurance review, and the money and time spent by hospitals in attracting and retaining physicians. Among the key attributes of transactions that influence their costliness are the uniqueness of the resources which each possesses (called asset specificity), uncertainty, and frequency of interaction. The more unique the resources involved, the greater the uncertainty, and the more frequent the interaction, the less costly it usually is to internalize the relationship than to deal through arm's length market transactions. These concepts are discussed in further depth subsequently.

It is also important to remember that the hospital-physician relationship takes place within the context of the doctor-patient relationship. The personal relationship between doctors and patients has been greatly altered by the changing organizational and economic climate of the 1980s. Prior to the 1980s, organizations primarily existed to service the doctor-patient relationship. The dominant tie was between the doctor and patient, both of whom had looser secondary ties to health care organizations. This has been altered in the 1980s as physicians and even patients have stronger ties with organizations that play a more dominant role in influencing what happens between the doctor and the patient (Sheldon 1986; Miller 1983).

ECONOMICS-BASED PERSPECTIVES

Buyer-Seller Relationship

In the economics-based perspective, physicians are viewed as purchasers or "demanders" (Harris 1977) of hospital services, while hospitals are viewed as the sellers or "suppliers." Thus, physicians constitute the "demand organization," particularly as reflected through the medical staff organization, while nursing and the various hospital ancillary support functions constitute the "supply organization." Under this perspective, the hospital's primary mission is to meet the needs of the buyers (i.e., the demanding physicians). To help assure that this occurs, the buyers organize themselves into a cooperative represented by the medical staff organization structure (Pauly and Redisch 1973). This model is most consistent with the physician-controlled era of the 1930–1974 period noted in Chapter 1. The changes that have occurred in the succeeding years, however, have posed a distinct threat to this concept of the relationship since they have significantly changed the hospitals' financial ability to meet physician demands on the one hand and, on the other hand, have given rise to multiple groups of new buyers (employers, consumer groups, and managed care purchasers) to whom attention must be paid.

Under the buyer-seller model, the medical staff organization was a useful mechanism for minimizing the transaction costs on the part of both hospitals and physicians. Hospitals faced accreditation and legal responsibilities that required physician input and oversight in reviewing the quality of patient care. These needs were met through the credentials committee and various medical audit and utilization review committees through which physicians voluntarily gave their time as part of the obligations associated with hospital privileges. Physicians, in turn, minimized their transaction costs by sharing among themselves the responsibility for overseeing quality assurance activities. The medical staff also served as a useful mechanism for organizing referrals in support of the physician's private practice (Shortell 1973; Burns and Wholey 1989).

The physician-hospital relationship, however, is a special type of buyer-seller relationship because of the seller's (i.e., the hospital's) role in overseeing much of the patient care activity that has been "purchased." Once the purchase has been made, the buyer normally takes responsibility for this activity (Teece 1987). The physician as buyer, however, essentially delegates much of this responsibility to the hospital, enabling physicians to maintain their autonomy and pursue other income-producing activities in their offices. The hospital's role is essentially that of an assembler of quality. Physicians maintain some control over the process through the medical staff organization functions and activities described above, which also helps to reduce the transaction costs for the hospital. The transaction costs between the hospital and physician can be further reduced through such mechanisms as employing full-time or part-time salaried medical directors or executive vice presidents for medical affairs, and through part-time or full-time salaried chiefs of service. To the extent that hospitals and physicians are complementary products, it is in the hospital's interest to align physicians as closely as possible to the hospital in order to improve the hospital's position vis-à-vis other purchasers of care and to further differentiate itself from competitors (Porter 1985, 418). Examples of these effects are discussed further in Chapter 12 (Joint Ventures) and Chapter 17 (Strengthening the Relationship).

Principal-Agent Relationship

An agent is someone who acts on behalf of or in place of another (the principal). In the doctor-patient relationship, the doctor is the agent acting on behalf of the patient. But in the hospital-physician relationship, the determination of who is the principal and who is the agent may vary. If the physician is viewed as the buyer and the hospital the supplier, then the hospital is the physician's agent in, for example, negotiating to obtain discounts on supplies or in purchasing major new technology. From this perspective, it is easy to understand physicians' anger when the hospital does things that appear to be competitive or contrary to physician desires (see Chapter 10). The hospital as agent is viewed as not acting in the principal's best interest. It is not simply an economic issue but a betrayal of trust.

In other situations, physicians may be viewed as agents acting on behalf of the hospital, as in the earlier noted case of providing emergency room coverage. From this perspective, any physician behavior that runs counter to hospital interests is viewed by the hospital as not only competitive but also reflecting a breach of trust. This perspective places the physician in the position of facing a double agent problem (Veatch 1983, 143). As the patient's agent, the physician's goal is to use whatever resources are needed to restore the patient to health. But as the agent for the hospital, the goal is to limit the amount of resources needed to restore the patient to health as expressed through conservative testing and early hospital discharge (Eisenberg 1986). While conserving resources and providing quality patient care are not inherently incompatible, they place increased strain on the hospital-physician relationship. As will be seen, this has resulted in the better hospitals searching for organizational integrative mechanisms for resolving the double agent problem while maintaining and even enhancing the viability of the institution.

Of particular interest is to consider the hospital's medical staff executive committee as the representative or agent of the staff physicians. Staff expects that the executive committee will fairly represent physician interests and take action to support their professional autonomy and values. On the other hand, the executive committee may be viewed by the hospital as an agent of its interests, thus presenting the executive committee with a different version of the classic double agent problem noted above. The problem, of course, is frequently more complicated than this since physicians have multiple and often conflicting interests, making it nearly impossible for the executive committee to speak with a united voice or represent all viewpoints equally well. Approaches for dealing with these issues are discussed in Part II (see especially Chapters 5 and 8).

ORGANIZATION-BASED PERSPECTIVE

In the organization-based perspective, hospitals and physicians are viewed as two relatively loosely coupled entities with different goals and objectives but with some interdependent needs. This relationship has been variously described as resulting in a dual hierarchy (Smith 1955), a heteronomous organization (Scott 1982), or an incompletely designed organization (Shortell 1985). As expressed by Friedson (1970, 175), "The profession constitutes a continuous breach in the walls of the organization." Whether the economic or legal form of the relationship is conceived of as buyer-seller or principal-agent is immaterial to the fact that organizational problems are created. These primarily involve coordinating work, managing conflicting interests, and setting strategic direction. As noted in Chapter 1, these problems have become particularly severe since 1974 due to increased managerial control of hospitals and of health care delivery at large.

Organization theorists also offer proposals or models for dealing with the problems. These center on mutual involvement and sharing of power and authority, variously described as a conjoint model (Scott 1982), shared authority (Shortell 1985), and professional bureaucracy (Mintzberg 1979; Schneller and Hughes 1988). This approach requires the willingness of both parties to give up something in the present to gain a potential desired good in the future. Hospital executives must be willing to give up or share some of the authority and control that they have gained in recent years, and physicians must be willing to give up some practice time and professional autonomy. The reward to be gained in the future is organizational and professional success—to position both the hospital and physician as the preferred providers of health care in their communities. Because the rewards are in the future and not immediate, creating the incentives for such a change is difficult. For the most part, deeply rooted cultural changes must take place. Both parties must let go of beliefs, attitudes, and behaviors that have been a source of satisfaction and pride in the past to adopt new beliefs, attitudes, and behaviors that, if not opposite to the original, are at the very least foreign.

THE ROLE OF TRANSACTION COSTS

Hospital-physician relationships are heavily influenced by the nature of the transaction costs incurred by each party. As previously noted, these costs are largely determined by the nature of asset specificity, behavioral and environmental uncertainty, and the frequency of interaction associated with the relationship. The more specific or unique (in the sense of not being able to be used for other purposes) the investments that the hospital as supplier must make to attract physicians, the greater the degree of physician commitment that hospitals will demand. Examples include investments in centers of excellence requiring considerable resources, such as those associated with heart transplantation and magnetic resonance imaging.

Uncertainty has two components: behavioral and environmental. Behavioral uncertainty refers to the predictability of response on the part of both the physician and the hospital. For example, from the hospital's perspective there is a great deal of behavioral uncertainty in working with physicians who have multiple hospital appointments and divided allegiances. From the perspective of physicians, behavioral uncertainty is involved in working with a hospital that has frequent CEO turnover. Environmental uncertainty refers to the lack of predictability due to such external factors as changes in regulations, third party payment, and general economic conditions. The greater the behavioral uncertainty involved, the greater the extent to which hospitals and physicians will approach each other cautiously and demand more guarantees in the relationship. The greater the environmental uncertainty involved, the greater the extent to which both hospitals and physicians will insist on provisions in the relationship that will buffer them from the uncertainty. Subsequent chapters dealing with managed care (Chapter 11) and joint ventures (Chapter 12) serve as examples.

As the frequency of interaction increases, the importance and cost of the relationship also increase. Thus, where transactions are expected to be frequent, more will be demanded by each party of the other. This is one reason why high admitting physicians are the most likely candidates for joint venture opportunities.

The transaction cost perspective, however, provides an incomplete understanding of hospital-physician relationships. It is also necessary to consider the benefits from an overall exchange perspective. This involves taking into account the strategic intent of both parties (Zajac and Olson 1989). Specifically, what does the hospital intend to achieve in its relationships with physicians, and vice versa? Thus, the overall relationship will be influenced by both the costs and benefits involved relative to the costs and benefits of other options available to each party.

From the hospital's perspective, the ultimate in reducing transaction costs lies in employing physicians on salary. Examples include the executive vice president for medical affairs, a full-time director of medical education, and paid section chiefs. Less complete approaches include restricting privileges to cost-effective providers (Glandon and Morrisey 1986), engaging in selected joint ventures, requiring longer terms of office for medical staff leaders to promote continuity and increase predictability of behavior, and increasing physician participation in the overall governance and management of the institution (Alexander, Morrisey, and Shortell 1986; Burns, Andersen, and Shortell 1989). A continuum of transaction cost–reducing mechanisms is shown in Figure 2.1. These mechanisms can also be viewed as reducing transaction costs from the physicians' perspective, but this depends on how important physicians believe the hospital is to their practice and the loss of autonomy involved in conducting such transactions relative to the benefits. Thus, from a transaction cost–benefit exchange perspective, it is not surprising to observe that the leadership in many hospital medical staffs is provided by the specialists and subspecialists for whom reducing the costs and increasing the benefits are most salient.

Figure 2.1 Transaction Cost–Reducing Mechanisms

LOW CHANGE					HIGH CHANGE
Education and appeal to over-arching goal or vision	Current medical staff organ-ization structure	More stringent specifica-tion of admitting priviliges and criteria for renewal of privileges	Parallel organiza-tion (e.g., physician-hospital or-ganization)	50-50 economic joint ventures	Hospital-employed physicians

THE CHANGING HEALTH CARE ENVIRONMENT

The changing health care environment, as highlighted in Chapter 1, is redefining the hospital-physician relationship by changing the nature of the transaction costs and benefits as viewed by both parties. Fixed payment rates, increased standards for evaluating quality of care, growing competition, and advances in technology have each placed great strain on using the traditional medical staff organization as the fulcrum for negotiating the relationship. Increased competition among physicians and specialty differences have made it increasingly difficult for the medical staff leaders to adequately represent physician views. The medical staff organization was never established to deal with the transaction costs and benefits of working out the economic business arrangements necessary for hospital and physician success in the new health care environment. As a result, there is a search for a new way of structuring the relationship with some examples shown on the continuum in Figure 2.2. The far left represents more or less the status quo but with attempts made to reduce the transaction costs by initiating greater continuity of medical staff leadership and more involvement of physicians in the overall management and governance of the institution. The expectation is that these efforts might improve the internal coordination, communication, conflict management, and problem-solving approaches of the organization—trouble spots which can increase internal transaction costs (Mick and Conrad 1988).

Moving to the middle of the continuum, one observes a variety of parallel organizational models or relationships (Shortell 1985) such as independent practice associations (IPAs), professional practice associations (PPAs), or joint physician-hospital organizations (PHOs). These relationships are attempts to get around the increasingly high costs of

Figure 2.2   A Continuum of Hospital-Physician Group Relationships

MODIFIED STATUS QUO	PARALLEL RELATIONSHIPS	CONTRACTUAL NEGOTIATIONS
Traditional relationship centered on hospital medical staff organization but with greater continuity of physician leadership and greater physician involvement in hospital management and governance	Development of parallel structures which coexist along with the hospital medical staff organization; the parallel structures primarily deal with economic relationships (IPAs, PPAs, PHOs, etc.)	Separate hospital and physician organizations; may be united through a health care plan or similar structure to provide care (e.g., Kaiser)

LEAST CHANGE	INTERMEDIATE CHANGE	MOST CHANGE

$\longrightarrow$

trying to transact such business through the medical staff organization structure by establishing new organizations specifically designed for contracting with outside parties or meeting the specific interests and needs of subgroups of physicians, for example, through joint ventures. While not without problems (as will be discussed in subsequent chapters), they are an attempt to increase the benefits to be gained by each party while reducing the internal organizational costs associated with negotiating contracts and monitoring behavior.

The far right represents the example of an arm's length independent contractual relationship between the hospital and a physician group. Rather than attempting to integrate physicians more fully into the current hospital structure, it allows physicians to develop their own independent organizational structure, such as in a multispecialty group practice or network of such practices, with their own goals and objectives, rewards and incentives, decision making, and control processes. A hospital and physician group then negotiate the contractual terms of the relationship involving the reciprocal services and responsibilities that each provides and receives. The closeness or tightness of the relationship can vary from an exclusive contract between a single hospital and physician group, as in the case of the Kaiser HMO model, to a looser relationship, which might be reflected in a hospital having contracts with several physician groups in the area. Likewise, a given physician group may have contracts with several hospitals. As previously noted, the form that the relationship takes will depend largely on the degree of asset specificity required by each party, the behavioral and environmental uncertainties experienced by each party, and the frequency of interaction required. The greater the asset specificity, the greater the behavioral and environmental uncertainty, and the greater the frequency of interaction demanded, the greater will be the incentives for an exclusive contractual relationship.

What is significant about the continuum shown in Figure 2.2 is that movement to the right results in a redefinition of the hospital-physician relationship away from the acute inpatient care institution and toward the other multiple settings in which health care will be delivered in the 1990s. Some of the present parallel structures (IPAs, PHOs, etc.) are best viewed as transitory organizations that will evolve toward contractual arrangements and new forms of reintegration. Hospitals will play an important role in these arrangements and in the larger delivery system, but it will not be based on the hospital's acute inpatient care expertise. Instead, it will be based on the hospital's ability to work with physicians and other health care professionals in putting together a delivery system that adds value for consumers in the local community. In making this transition, it is important to realize that the nature of the buyer-seller relationship and the principal-agent relationship may change as new conjoint or shared models are developed to meet the new demands. Some glimpses of what these relationships may look like, along with some guidelines for managing them successfully, are examined in subsequent chapters. Many of the guidelines and lessons described can be viewed as attempts by the study sites to reduce the transaction costs and increase the mutual benefits that might be associated with various partnership arrangements.

REFERENCES

Alexander, J. A., M. A. Morrisey, and S. M. Shortell. 1986. "The Effects of Competition, Regulation and Corporatization on Hospital-Physician Relationships," *Journal Health and Social Behavior* 27:220–35.

Burns, L. R., R. M. Andersen, and S. M. Shortell. 1989. "The Impact of Corporate Structures on Physician Inclusion and Participation," *Medical Care* 27 (10):967–82.

Burns, L. R., and D. R. Wholey. 1989. "Determinants of Organizational Commitment among Professionals: A Longitudinal Analysis of Physician Exit and Loyalty," College of Business and Public Administration, University of Arizona, August.

Eisenberg, J. M. 1986. *Doctors' Decisions and the Cost of Medical Care.* Ann Arbor, MI: Health Administration Press Perspectives.

Fama, E., and M. C. Jensen. 1986. "Agency Problems and Residual Claims," *Journal of Law and Economics* 26:327–49.

Friedson, E. 1970. *Professional Dominance.* Chicago: Aldine.

Glandon, G. L., and M. A. Morrisey. 1986. "Redefining the Hospital-Physician Relationship under Prospective Payment," *Inquiry* 23(Summer):175–86.

Harris, J. E. 1977. "The Internal Organization of Hospitals: Some Economic Implications," *Bell Journal of Economics* 8:467–82.

Mick, S. S., and D. A. Conrad. 1988. "The Decision to Integrate Vertically in Health Care Organizations," *Journal of Hospital and Health Services Administration* 33:345–60.

Miller, F. H. 1983. "Secondary Income from Recommended Treatment: Should Fiduciary Relationships Constrain Physician Behavior?" in B. Gray (Ed.), *The New Health Care For Profit*. Washington, DC: National Academy of Sciences Press, Institute of Medicine, 153–69.

Mintzberg, H. 1979. *The Structuring of Organizations*. Englewood Cliffs, NJ: Prentice-Hall.

Newhouse, J. P. 1970. "Toward a Theory of Nonprofit Institutions: An Economic Model of a Hospital," *American Economic Review* 60:64.

Pauly, M. V. 1980. *Doctors and Their Workshops: Economic Models of Physician Behavior*. Chicago: University of Chicago Press.

Pauly, M. V., and M. Redisch. 1973. "The Not-for-Profit Hospital as Physician's Cooperative," *The American Economic Review*, 63(March):87–100.

Porter, M. E. 1985. *Competitive Advantage*. New York: Macmillan.

Schneller, E. S., and R. G. Hughes. 1988. "The Future of Medicine," in R. Schenke (Ed.), *The Physician in Management*. 2nd ed. Tampa, FL: American Academy of Medical Directors, 22–43.

Scott, W. R. 1982. "Managing Professional Work: Three Models of Control for Health Organizations," *Health Services Research* 17:213–40.

Sheldon, A. 1986. *Managing Doctors*. Homewood, IL: Dow Jones–Irwin.

Shortell, S. M. 1973. "Patterns of Referral Among Internists in Private Practice: A Social Exchange Model," *Journal of Health and Social Behavior* (December): 335–48.

———. 1985. "The Medical Staff of the Future: Replanting the Garden," *Frontiers of Health Services Management* 1:3–48.

Smith, H. L. 1955. "Two Lines of Authority Are One Too Many," *Modern Hospital* (March):84.

Teece, D. J., Ed. 1987. *The Competitive Challenge: Strategies for Industrial Innovation and Renewal*. Cambridge, MA: Ballinger.

Veatch, R. M. 1983. "Ethical Dilemmas of For-Profit Enterprise in Health Care," in B. Gray (Ed.), *The New Health Care For Profit: Doctors and Hospitals in a Competitive Environment*. Washington, DC: Institute of Medicine, National Academy of Sciences, 125–52.

Williamson, O. 1975. *Markets and Hierarchies: Analysis and Antitrust Implications*. New York: The Free Press.

———. 1985. *The Economic Institutions of Capitalism: Firms, Markets, and Relational Contracting*. New York: The Free Press.

Zajac, E., and C. Olsen. 1989. "From Transaction Costs to Transactional Analysis: Implications for the Study of Interorganizational Strategies." Paper presented at the Ninth Annual Strategic Management Society Conference, San Francisco.

CHAPTER 3

Study Design

SAMPLE SELECTION

The primary focus of the study was on not-for-profit and investor-owned community general hospitals. Major medical center affiliated or owned teaching hospitals were excluded because much is already known about the primarily salaried relationships at these institutions and the divisional model of organization used by Johns Hopkins and others (Heyssel 1984). Major selection criteria included geography, bed size, ownership, freestanding versus system hospitals, and degree of teaching activity. With these criteria in mind, approximately 40 hospitals believed to have effective hospital-physician relationships were identified by a nine-member advisory committee (of physician, executive, and association experts) in consultation with other leaders in the field.[1] After further discussion, the list was reduced to approximately 25 institutions, who were then called for further information and verification of the nature of the relationship between the hospital and its physicians. Based on this information, 10 institutions were asked to participate in the study; due to time constraints, 2 declined and were replaced by 2 equivalent institutions.

The ten sites and their background characteristics are shown in Table 3.1; Tables 3.2 and 3.3 provide overall summaries. As shown in Table 3.2, the sites are well distributed geographically across the country with a balanced mix of freestanding and system hospitals, and teaching versus nonteaching institutions. One investor-owned hospital is represented. There is also a good mix in regard to employment of an executive vice president for medical affairs or medical director, full-time or part-time section chiefs, parallel organizations (for example, PHO, IPA), HMO/PPO sponsorship, and economic joint ventures with physicians. Interestingly, the majority of the sites have two-year terms of office for medical staff leaders rather than the more customary one-year term.

Table 3.1 Site Background Characteristics

Hospital Name and Location	Region	Ownership	Bed Size	Average Occupancy Rate 1985–1988 (%)	CEO Tenure (years)	Size of Active Staff	Active Staff Board Certified (%)	Active Staff with Two or More Appointments (%)	Number of Physicians Who are Voting Members of Governing Board
Catherine McAuley Health Center Ann Arbor, MI	Midwest	Not-for-profit system	554	83	13	401	75	75	3
Crouse-Irving Memorial Hospital Syracuse, NY	East	Not-for-profit freestanding	612	93	9	500	94	90	1
Leonard Morse Hospital Natick, MA	New England	Not-for-profit freestanding	259	67	4	95	82	80	1
Lexington Medical Center West Columbia, SC	South	Not-for-profit freestanding	292	78	1.5	166	82	80	3

North Monroe Hospital Monroe, LA	South	Investor-owned system	190	75	4	93	63	100	5
Providence Medical Center Seattle, WA	Northwest	Not-for-profit system	376	68	9	324	77	80	0
Scripps Memorial Hospital La Jolla, CA	West	Not-for-profit system	476	69	12	740	80	80	1
Sutter Community Hospitals* Sacramento, CA	West	Not-for-profit system	353	92	10	903	78	90	4
Tucson Medical Center Tucson, AZ	Southwest	Not-for-profit freestanding	615	63	23	428	90	100	4
West Allis Memorial West Allis, WI	Midwest	Not-for-profit freestanding	238	69	18	148	98	95	3

*Except for bedsize and occupancy rate, data reflect shared staff between Sutter Memorial and Sutter General.

Table 3.2   Site Selection Summary: General Background Characteristics

Region
　　2 East/New England
　　2 Midwest
　　2 South
　　1 Northwest
　　2 West
　　1 Southwest

Ownership
　　4 Not-for-profit system
　　5 Not-for-profit freestanding
　　1 Investor-owned system

Teaching Activity (i.e., House Staff)
　　6 Yes
　　4 No

Full- or Part-Time Medical Director or Executive V.P. for Medical Affairs
　　5 Yes
　　5 No

Full-Time or Part-Time Section Chiefs
　　3 Yes
　　7 No

Have a Parallel Organization (PHO, JV Corporation, IPA, etc.)
　　7 Yes
　　3 No

HMO/PPO Sponsorship
　　4 Yes
　　6 No

Economic Joint Ventures with Physicians
　　6 Yes
　　4 No

Two-Year Term of Office for Medical Staff Leaders
　　8 Yes
　　2 No

Table 3.3 indicates that the ten sites are larger in bed size than the national average and also have somewhat higher occupancy rates and profit margins. Seven of the ten sites were market leaders, and the remaining were among the leaders. They enjoyed a relatively high degree of CEO stability and had a higher percentage of active staff physicians who were board certified than the national average of approximately 66 percent (Musacchio et al. 1986). In brief, while not without challenges to face, the ten study hospitals are largely successful institutions. They were engaged in a number of important and interesting activities with their physicians and, therefore, served as a rich laboratory for learning about effective hospital-physician relationships.

DATA COLLECTION

A three-pronged approach to data collection was developed. First, background documents such as hospital strategic plans, annual reports, medical staff bylaws, and quality assurance plans were examined. This was followed by intensive two-day site visits involving structured interviews with an average of 14 persons per site. These included board chairmen, CEOs, chief operating officers, the vice president for nursing, medical staff leaders (including the executive vice president for medical affairs or medical director, section chiefs, and the president of the staff), the leader of a parallel organization such as an independent practice association or joint physician hospital organization, and at least one younger physician (under 40 years). The interviews averaged 1 to 1½ hours in length and covered topics related to the history and background of the relationship; the perceived strengths and weaknesses of the relationship; accomplishments and problems; issues of trust, communication, and methods of conflict resolution; physician involvement in decision making; a number of specific issues related to credentialing, hospital-physician competition, managed care contracting, joint ventures, physician-nurse relationships, and quality assurance; and plans for the future (see Appendix A for a copy of the interview instrument).

Table 3.3 Site Selection Summary: Operational Characteristics

	Mean	*Range*
Bed size	379	190–615
Occupancy rate (1985–1988)	73.4	63–94
Operating Margin* (1985–1988)	3.61	−0.94–8.0
CEO tenure	10.5	1.5–23
Active staff size	324	93–735
Percent of active staff board certified	81.7	63–98
Percent of active staff with two or more hospital appointments	87	75–100
Number of physicians who are voting members of the governing board	2.3	0–5

*Operating Margin = $\dfrac{\text{Net operating income}}{\text{Revenue from patient care operations only}}$

Overall, 138 interviews were conducted involving 89 physicians, 37 hospital executives, and 12 board members (some of the physicians and executives were also board members). During the visit, minutes of the most recent year's board of directors meetings and the medical staff executive committee meetings were abstracted. This information was used to help verify interview data and provide leads for additional questions regarding key events (see Appendix A for the abstracting form).

A third source of information was a 70-item self-administered questionnaire completed by each person interviewed prior to the visit. The questionnaire addressed a number of issues related to various aspects of the hospital-physician relationship, such as the degree of hospital support of physicians; leadership, teamwork, and decision-making issues; admission policies; hospital-physician competition; physician recruitment; physician autonomy, and related issues (see Appendices A and B). All of the data and information derived from the above sources were updated and further elaborated as a result of a follow-up symposium in which representatives from nine of the ten institutions shared their experiences and future plans for strengthening the hospital-physician relationship.

ANALYSIS

Based on prior research and experience, the framework shown in Figure 3.1 was used to guide the data collection and subsequent analysis. Beginning on the right, the effectiveness of the hospital-physician relationship was viewed as a function of how well they interact with each other in regard to such issues as the degree of trust established, effectiveness of communication, dealing with conflict, and managing change. In order to obtain an in-depth understanding of these processes, a set of "relationship tracers" was used involving salient and frequently occurring issues. As shown, these included physician credentialing and disciplining, physician recruitment, hospital-physician competition, joint ventures, and quality assurance, among others. The far left portion of the figure illustrates that how these issues are handled and the process dynamics associated with them will be influenced by the external environment facing both hospitals and physicians, the leadership styles and decision-making skills of those involved, hospital strategies, various structural and process factors, and the organization's history and culture.

All interviews were transcribed verbatim and then categorized by respondent name, hospital name, respondent position, and the question/topic number corresponding to specific issues such as trust or con-

Figure 3.1 Guiding Conceptual Framework for Studying Effective Hospital-Physician Relationships

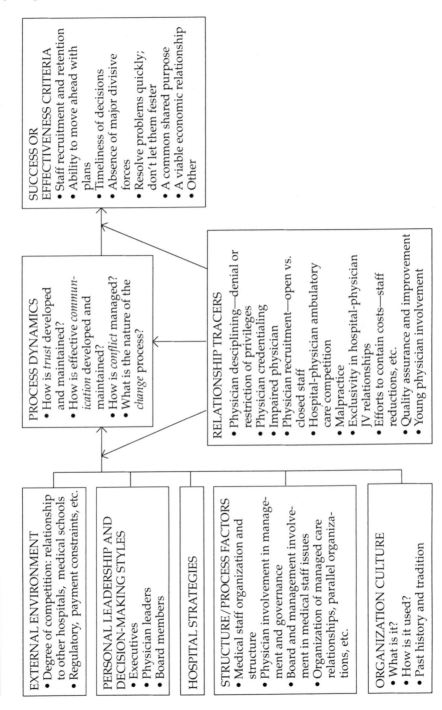

SUCCESS OR
EFFECTIVENESS CRITERIA
- Staff recruitment and retention
- Ability to move ahead with plans
- Timeliness of decisions
- Absence of major divisive forces
- Resolve problems quickly; don't let them fester
- A common shared purpose
- A viable economic relationship
- Other

PROCESS DYNAMICS
- How is *trust* developed and maintained?
- How is effective *communication* developed and maintained?
- How is *conflict* managed?
- What is the nature of the *change* process?

RELATIONSHIP TRACERS
- Physician disciplining—denial or restriction of privileges
- Physician credentialing
- Impaired physician
- Physician recruitment—open vs. closed staff
- Hospital-physician ambulatory care competition
- Malpractice
- Exclusivity in hospital-physician JV relationships
- Efforts to contain costs—staff reductions, etc.
- Quality assurance and improvement
- Young physician involvement

EXTERNAL ENVIRONMENT
- Degree of competition: relationship to other hospitals, medical schools
- Regulatory, payment constraints, etc.

PERSONAL LEADERSHIP AND
DECISION-MAKING STYLES
- Executives
- Physician leaders
- Board members

HOSPITAL STRATEGIES

STRUCTURE/PROCESS FACTORS
- Medical staff organization and structure
- Physician involvement in management and governance
- Board and management involvement in medical staff issues
- Organization of managed care relationships, parallel organizations, etc.

ORGANIZATION CULTURE
- What is it?
- How is it used?
- Past history and tradition

flict management (Miles and Huberman 1984; Levine 1985; Weinholtz and Friedman 1985). In order to determine whether a specific statement or response reflected a specific topic of interest (for example, a statement about a joint venture issue versus a cost containment issue or a statement involving decision-making style versus organizational culture), the principal investigator and a doctoral student research assistant independently content-analyzed 28 interviews involving 1,000 passages from the first five sites visited. The overall level of agreement between the two raters was 84.8 percent, with a range across sites from 78.6 to 90 percent. Most differences were resolved through further discussion. Those that remained confusing were deleted from consideration as directly quotable material or as representing a clear example of one issue versus another.

Analyses were conducted both across issues within each site as well as across sites within each issue. The former approach permits each site to be viewed as a whole (Ragin 1987), taking into account how the various issues and factors interact with each other in influencing relationships at that site. The latter approach permits one to examine how the issues and factors operate across sites. How prevalent are the various issues? What are the commonalties and differences? Because the purpose of this book is to develop lessons and guidelines that cut across sites, greater emphasis is given to the second approach; hence, the organization of the book is by topic or issue rather than by individual chapters for each site. For a more holistic perspective on each site, see the material in Appendix C.

Having established the reliability and validity of the categorization of the interview material, each interview was read in its entirety and summaries of the most frequently occurring problems, accomplishments, issues, best practices, strengths, weaknesses, and so on were developed for each site and then aggregated across sites. Analyses were also done to see if physician responses differed from board members and hospital executives. With the exception of the perception of accomplishments and, to a lesser extent, criteria for judging effectiveness, there were no systematic differences between the physician respondents and the hospital executives and board members. The differences noted are discussed in subsequent sections.

Overall impressions obtained during the site visits were also summarized, along with key data gleaned from the background material and the summary of board and medical staff executive committee minutes. This approach helped to identify the more important and frequently occurring issues, challenges, approaches, and success stories. These form the substance of the remaining chapters.

NOTE

1. The 40 hospitals (including the subset of 10 eventually selected) do not constitute a representative sample of the nation's hospitals. Neither are they the only hospitals that may have earned reputations for having particularly effective hospital-physician relationships. On the whole, however, they proved to be worthy and instructive sites for examining the issues addressed by the study.

REFERENCES

Heyssel, R. M. 1984. "Decentralized Management in a Teaching Hospital," *The New England Journal of Medicine* 310(22):1477–80.

Levine, H. G. 1985. "Principles of Data Storage and Retrieval for Use in Qualitative Evaluations," *Educational Evaluation and Policy Analysis* 7(2):169–86.

Miles, M. B. and A. M. Huberman. 1984. *Qualitative Data Analysis: A Sourcebook of New Methods.* Beverly Hills, CA: Sage Publications.

Musacchio, R. A., S. Zuckerman, L. E. Jensen, and L. Freshnock. 1986. "Hospital Ownership and the Practice of Medicine: Evidence from the Physician's Perspective" in B. Gray (Ed.), *For-Profit Enterprise in Health Care.* Washington, DC: National Academy Press, Institute of Medicine, 385–401.

Ragin, C. C. 1987. *The Comparative Method: Moving Beyond Quantitative and Qualitative Strategies.* Berkeley: University of California Press.

Weinholtz, D., and C. P. Friedman. 1985. "Conducting Qualitative Studies Using Theory and Previous Research: A Study Re-examined," *Evaluation and the Health Professions* 8(2):149–76.

PART II

Managing the Relationship

CHAPTER 4

Defining an Effective Relationship

While there is vast literature on organizational effectiveness (Scott and Shortell 1988), there is almost none that examines the effectiveness of specific relationships in which the overall relationship itself is the unit of analysis, apart from the outcomes of specific bargaining, negotiation, or conflict situations. Therefore, before examining the factors associated with effective hospital-physician relationships, it is necessary to define what is meant by an effective relationship. Analyses indicated that respondents use two major dimensions—process criteria and outcome criteria—as shown in Table 4.1. Each is highlighted below.

PROCESS CRITERIA

When physicians, hospital executives, and board members think about the effectiveness of their relationship, they think about the daily process of interactions among themselves as much as they do about the outcome of these interactions. Particularly important to them are frequent, honest, and open communication, and the ability to tackle issues together, to move on things, and to address problems in a timely fashion. The following statements are illustrative. By a McAuley physician board member:

> I have a framework that I use and that framework says if there's not a level of rapport, we'll never achieve understanding. . . . It goes beyond just some of the social ties; it's a fundamental issue of looking across the table and knowing that there's a level of mutual respect, but more fundamentally the issue of trust. . . . I think if you have rapport, then you can achieve a level of understanding. . . . In many ways it's an issue of what information are you sharing in common.

One of the things that I've learned recently is to depoliticize issues and to move them out of being where the warfarer has waged his own opinions. In order to be constructive one needs to move to the place where credible information is being brought forth that both groups can see and buy into. . . .

Then the last stage is the willingness to mutually defend our agreements, which means coming back and saying to a surgeon or doctor, my understanding is this. We came to this level of agreement. Unless I've missed the point some place, what happened, happened because I need to defend this agreement. A lot of it for me is very much on an informal basis with each physician, with groups of physicians, and then as I'm rewriting contracts, working that out so that we have frameworks that we can look at each other and go back to a common level of understanding.

A North Monroe physician commented:

Personally, I think the key to it is the openness of communication, the reception which administration gives to physician ideas. I think both have a common goal, and when each perceives that goal as their common interest, there's no problem, and that's been true here. And I contrast that with [a competing hospital] where there's

Table 4.1   Criteria for Evaluating the Effectiveness of the Hospital-
Physician Relationship

Process Criteria

Frequent, open, honest communication

Ability to move on things together; tackle the tough issues

Extent to which problems are addressed in an effective and timely fashion

Extent and quality of physician involvement and participation (in strategic planning, committee work, volunteer activities)

A reasonably low level of complaints; good morale

Outcome Criteria

Patient admissions, occupancy rate, market share

Physician recruitment and retention

Quality of care that physicians practice

Adherence to standards of accountability

Collaborative and successful hospital-physician joint ventures been a very distant relationship. What's good for the hospital is not necessarily good for the patients or the physicians. . . . I think it is a real compliment to this administration in that no matter what the problem, it was the patient's well-being that counted. And physicians appreciate that, so it has been a very warm and cooperative relationship here.

A Scripps hospital executive noted:

We have a lot of forums. We meet with our chief of staff regularly. I try and spend a lot of time in the surgeons' or doctors' lounge, going in and having a cup of coffee in the morning, and I'll always walk out with one or two agenda items. We try to increase our visibility. We're all around at least one day a week, and it's to the point if I don't do it on a Wednesday, then I've penalized myself and I do it on Saturday morning. . . . We also go overboard in communicating with employees. I learned early on that something I say to employees will end up being quoted by physicians in a committee meeting and they don't even know it came from me. There is a lot of communication going on between our nurses and physicians. . . . It's interesting how the information flows back to the medical staff very rapidly.

The extent and quality of physician involvement and overall morale are also key factors. The physician's perspective on these issues is highlighted by a McAuley physician:

Physicians look at how responsive the hospital is to their concerns and needs. Does the hospital really listen? Do they understand our problems, and what are they doing to help solve those problems? If the hospital has a program or has a proposed way of dealing with an issue and the medical staff has concerns about it, does the hospital really listen to the physicians and modify that program to accommodate or to help accommodate some of the concerns or all of the concerns that the medical staff might have? Or is it "we can talk about it but the decision is already made" type of approach? That's the question.

In a similar fashion, a Tucson physician noted:

Unrest in the staff. The guy stops you in the halls and says, hey, I don't know why we are doing this, or what the hell is going on, or hey, I don't like this. I don't hear so much of that, because I think they are better informed because we have more physicians involved at both the board level and the financial level.

OUTCOME CRITERIA

Those interviewed were also realists in recognizing that the ultimate test of the relationship was whether it was enabling hospitals and physicians to meet their objectives. These included both economic objectives related to patient admissions, market share, and successful joint ventures and objectives reflecting professional values involving the quality of care provided and meeting standards of accountability. A North Monroe executive noted:

> I think that we're continuing to move forward, to meet our objectives and the goals that we have established. When you're a 110-bed hospital and you're taking on a 400-bed tertiary care facility and some other community hospitals, you've got to have a strategic plan in place, and recognize you're not going to compete service for service. You've got to build on your medical staff; you've got to develop market niches where you can develop centers of excellence where you become superior. The strategic plan becomes very critical. I guess I measure where we're at in terms of what have we successfully completed in that plan and where we're at in that plan.

A Providence executive noted:

> The relationship needs to permit accomplishment of economic objectives and managed care systems. Involvement in managed care systems, other kinds of practice and systems of physicians that need to be successful. The hospital has to have its medical staff succeed in order for it to succeed. A relationship is needed that allows the hospital to use its resources and wherewithal to help a physician succeed. I think it opens up all kinds of ventures, the office building, the clinics, and we also have primary care groups that are employed in those clinics, and we have rotating specialists who are good for the clinics. We can get our specialists there in a way that works. [It gives us] the ability to accomplish what needs to be accomplished in those areas.

A Tucson executive commented:

> We track the total market share discharges of physicians, and we know over a two-year period, by six-month increments, what percentage of market share a physician is bringing to Tucson Medical Center of his total cases. And I was sitting here yesterday afternoon with a physician that in the last six months of '87 was bringing 50 percent of his patients here. In the first six months of '88 he

was bringing 28 percent. And he was in here telling us he'd like to do more with Tucson Medical Center. And I say, yeah, but the record here shows that you have done less. Well, we should be able to spot problems, not only in the decline but in the increase that certain physicians bring to us.

A Lexington board member commented:

One of the things we use is quality assurance indicators. Are the physicians doing their job? Are they accountable? Are they facing up to their problems?

HOSPITAL VERSUS PHYSICIAN RESPONDENTS

For half the sites, the effectiveness criteria mentioned by board members and hospital executives were similar to those mentioned by physicians. For the other five sites, the physicians more frequently mentioned such factors as

1. the receptiveness of the hospital to physician ideas
2. the ability and willingness of the hospital to provide up-to-date technology
3. the general accessibility of hospital administration to the physicians
4. the lack of competitive relationships between the hospital and its physicians

SUMMARY

The process and outcome criteria examined here are generally consistent with those developed by a physician leadership task force of the Voluntary Hospitals of America (1988). Their criteria included

1. a mutuality of interest with a common shared purpose
2. the ability to respond to community needs
3. a viable economic relationship that can respond to buyers' requirements
4. continuity of medical staff leadership
5. a disciplined organized medical staff capable of responding as a unit
6. an ability to learn and incorporate new information into ongoing decision making

These, then, are the criteria by which hospitals and physicians evaluate the effectiveness of their relationship. They involve both process and outcomes, but the study participants saw a very close relationship between the two. A hospital's financial viability and ability to meet community need and market demands depended importantly on their ability to recruit and retain high-quality physicians with whom they could pursue opportunities of mutual interest. This, in turn, depended importantly on the quality of physician involvement in the institution, the quality of communication, and the ability to address problems in a timely and effective fashion and to move forward on issues of importance. The specific ways in which these criteria were met are taken up in the following chapters, beginning with a discussion of managerial style, decision-making approaches, and physician involvement.

REFERENCES

Scott, W. R., and S. M. Shortell. 1988. "Organizational Performance: Managing For Efficiency and Effectiveness," in S. M. Shortell and A. D. Kaluzny (Eds.), *Healthcare Management: A Text in Organization Theory and Behavior*. New York: John Wiley, 418–57.

Voluntary Hospitals of America. 1988. Physician Task Force Meeting, Irving, Texas, May, 1988.

CHAPTER 5

Managerial Style, Decision-Making Approaches, and Physician Involvement

INTRODUCTION

The process by which decisions are made serves as an important lens for examining the hospital-physician relationship. As previously noted, this process is becoming increasingly complex as hospitals and physicians work to find an appropriate balance in the relationship. The degree of involvement, the timing of involvement, the importance of the issue, and the types of people to involve all affect the relationship. Research indicates that hospitals have generally increased all forms of physician involvement and integrating mechanisms (Alexander, Morrisey, and Shortell 1986), but the effects of these on the relationship is largely unexamined (for exceptions see Burns, Andersen, and Shortell 1989, 1990).

In the ten cases studied, the overall level of satisfaction with the degree of physician involvement in the decision-making process was outstanding in three cases, good in four cases, and mixed in the remaining three. The outstanding sites were distinguished from the merely good by the extent of physician ongoing involvement in the strategic planning process of the institution in addition to involvement in operational decisions affecting clinical practice. Other studies confirm that where physician involvement occurs, it is often in regard to operational issues affecting clinical practice rather than externally oriented strategic issues (McDaniel 1990). Where satisfaction with the degree of involvement was somewhat mixed, respondents felt the need to be more involved in the management and governance of the institution, particularly as reflected in the strategic planning process. They saw this process as beginning to directly influence operational decisions affecting their clinical autonomy and practice styles. This was particularly true for decisions involving nursing practices and policies. Lack of involvement in nursing practices and policies was the most frequently mentioned operational issue across nearly all sites. In contrast, most physicians at all sites were generally satisfied with their participation in decisions involving major allocations of capital and the purchase of new technology and equipment.

Many of these respondents, however, indicated that their views on participation and involvement were not necessarily shared by the medical staff at large. In the words of one: "You have to understand that we are really three groups—the management and board, the medical staff leadership, and the rank and file. For the most part, we [the medical staff leadership] are a lot closer to the management and board than we are to the rank and file." This view is expressed diagrammatically in Figure 5.1 and was largely confirmed in interviews with younger physicians constituting the staff at large. In some of the sites, there existed something close to what might be called a "rank and file" culture characterized by a general suspicion of the hospital as an institution, a wariness of medical staff leadership, and a "show me" attitude. Unless these physicians could see the relevance of a hospital or medical staff leadership decision for the physician's own practice and aspirations, apathy prevailed. If the decision was perceived to have a negative impact, open hostility was prevalent. There was little evidence of staff physicians *initiating* proposals to the hospital that might improve either their lot or the hospital's. Thus, a key lesson is the need for management and physician leaders to work with younger staff to develop a sense of interdependence and shared responsibility. As previously noted, in one case the situation became so acute that the staff at large attempted to oust the current medical staff leadership and set up their own structure. The challenge is also reflected by the experience of a non–study site in trying to establish a medical director position. The medical staff executive committee polled the staff at large and found that two-thirds of 150 responding physicians favored creation of a medical director position. At a subsequent meeting, however, the staff voted 67–59 to formally censure its own executive committee for proposing the position.

The bifurcation between medical staff leadership and the staff at large was, as expected, influenced by medical staff size (the larger the staff, the more difficulties reported). But it was also affected by processes of communication, conflict resolution, and levels of trust (discussed in subsequent chapters). Further, it was influenced in important ways by the history and culture of the organization, management stability, managerial leadership and decision-making style, and the quality of physician leadership (discussed in this chapter). The types, timing,

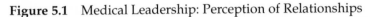

Figure 5.1 Medical Leadership: Perception of Relationships

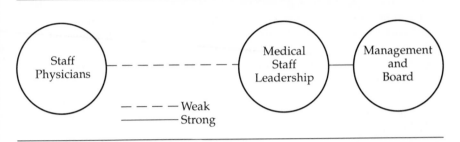

and levels of involvement are also examined, paying particular attention to the strategic planning process. Two minicases illustrate some key points, and some of the major lessons and guidelines are summarized as "best practices."

FACTORS INFLUENCING INVOLVEMENT

History and Culture

The histories and cultures of the organizations studied played an important role in influencing the extent and nature of physician involvement in decision making. Eight of the ten sites had a history and culture generally supportive of physician involvement. For some, such as McAuley Health Center, there was a long history dating back to 1911. For others, such as North Monroe and Lexington, a shorter history was involved dating from the 1970s. The situation at McAuley:

> An important factor going back many years was the fact that it was the physicians who asked the sisters to start the hospital. There has been a strong relationship between the management and the physicians. By that, I mean the physicians have been accepted as part of the team. There is no we/they attitude. Back in the '40s or earlier, the nuns who ran the hospital were very smart. They invited the physicians to have offices in the hospital. That was pretty unique for the time. For example, in the early '50s our strongest program here was cardiology. The reason for that is the nuns recruited physicians to come on board full-time and run that program. The director really determined how the program was going to be developed and had his office in the hospital. All of the clinical space was built within the hospital. It's pretty hard to hate the other guy

when you're walking by each other every day. The administrators' office was 200 feet from the clinic area where there were 15 physicians practicing. When you walked down to the lunchroom, you would walk by their offices; so there was a lot of interaction between the management and the medical staff. As a result, a key factor in our success is physician participation in decision making. We demand participation in decision making. It's kind of interesting because sometimes you will hear complaints about how we're too slow in our decision making. The reason for that is that we have a lot of participation. We're always looking for new people to get involved. The management team is really tuned in to looking for the young people coming up who would be good participants in decision making, who can assimilate information, and who have good conceptual skills.

The administration can build on such history and culture to foster positive physician involvement:

When I took this job 12 years ago, I think the management team had deteriorated somewhat in that we had several administrators who were pretty antagonistic towards physicians. So basically we cleaned out the management team, and we have consistently recruited people for the last 12 years who come into this place with a different attitude towards medical staff and physicians. We don't want people who are intimidated by physicians. They tend to end up resenting physicians. So we look for people that have a lot of self-confidence, who can deal with physicians as equals. They don't wilt in front of physicians. But they also treat them with respect, they respect their opinion, and they respect their intelligence. They understand that they have to be full participants if we're going to be successful. When I first became the CEO, there was concern that I was giving the hospital away to the doctors.

The hospital board can play a key role in helping to set the overall tone for the relationship. As expressed by the chairman of the board at West Allis:

We have cultivated physician involvement over the years. We [the board] are willing to learn. There are no "doctor haters" on the board.

A physician at Providence commented:

First of all, I have to say the administration and the sisters of Providence are committed to having a good relationship in communicating well with the medical staff. I also think that most of the physicians that practice here share a lot of the same values. It is always amazing when I talk with physicians at [another hospital], we just think differently. I mean they just don't think about the role of the hospital. If you talk to the doctors here they really appreciate what Providence is doing for them. So having shared values makes physicians a lot more willing and eager to work at the hospital.

An executive at Tucson Medical Center noted:

I think the strategy in the beginning of giving physicians more say as a collective group has helped. We've tried to treat all physicians alike. I'm not going to say that there aren't ways in which little favors get done informally, but essentially it's been one of trying to be fair. For example, if you want surgical time, it's on a first-come, first-served basis. . . . I think the teaching program here has also made a big difference in our success. It has cost us a bundle to be involved in medical education, but we've got value out of it because of the physicians we've been able to attract. They like to be in a teaching environment, but they don't want to be controlled by an academic medical staff. So I think we've attracted the best physicians here by having a teaching program.

Several other institutions also commented on the important role that medical education played in attracting qualified physicians and providing a solid foundation for involvement. Another Providence physician noted:

From my own personal point of view, I think a large number of people enjoy the relationship with the University of Washington. I think that's an important feature. While it has cost us something, it may in fact be necessary for our survival. Without it, I think some of the physicians would be gone.

A McAuley physician stated:

There's just a tremendous tradition in Ann Arbor with two major medical centers, and everybody here is very well trained and usually comes from a major medical center. A lot of people come from the University, and I think that all has a positive influence. A lot of people come here on staff who have been professors for a number of years, and that enhances everyone. You not only have good doctors, but you have a special group of people who have been involved in education and research which strengthens the institution.

Management Stability

Management stability was a second factor influencing physician involvement. Overall, in seven of the ten sites, the CEO, COO, and vice president for nursing had been in their position for at least eight years; in two sites, between three and seven years; and in only one site had one or more of these individuals been in their position for less than three years.

Stability of the top management team helped to promote a climate of physician involvement and supportive relationships in many ways. First, management stability helped to provide psychological security for physicians (and others) at a time when the environment encouraged so much insecurity and anxiety. As one CEO commented: "I think the physicians find it reassuring in knowing that we're still here." A related factor was the predictability that grew out of having a stable top management team. Both physicians and executives knew what to expect from each other. Issues could be anticipated and likely reactions discussed. Physicians knew how authority would be handled and how decisions would be made (Lang 1988). As one executive commented:

> Because we've all been here a while, they [the physicians] know what to expect from us. They know we won't surprise them. They trust us. On our part, we also know better what to expect from them. We know what we need to bring to them and what we don't. In a way we have more freedom and flexibility in our relationship because of this.

As hinted above, stability also gave each party greater knowledge of the other. This helped in addressing issues more quickly. It also helped in socializing new physicians regarding "how things are done around here" and in establishing the values and linkages to the past. As expressed by one corporate president:

> I waited a long time to turn this hospital over to [the current executive] because when he came here, he came as a department head and in about five years I said, this is the guy. If he keeps developing, then I want to do this. Because he was not only prepared, but he had a value system that was consistent. Don't expect us to agree on the professional management decisions. We will have disagreement on that. But I want some consistency in values. And throughout the organization, we've had continuity of top people. One has been here 14 years, another 21 years, another 25 years, and so on. As a result, we have good people that have a sense of caring and values that fit the culture of the organization, and I fight to protect it.

Management stability also heavily influenced the way in which problems were formulated and how conflicts were managed. When physicians were working with a management team that had been with the institution for years and was likely to continue to be with it for the foreseeable future, problems were more likely to be defined in terms of joint ownership (physician and hospital) rather just the hospital alone. They were likely to be defined as "our" problems, and not "theirs," because the history and experience of working together created a sense of interdependency. Differences and conflicts were more likely to be handled in open collaborative problem-solving approaches because each party knew they would have to continue to live with each other in the long run. As one vice president expressed it:

> It's like being married to each other. We feel free to say what's on our mind, but we also know we have to face each other tomorrow morning. We want the relationship to work in the long run, so we're pretty careful about maintaining mutual respect. As a result, there are fewer attempts to ram things down each other's throats.

Instead, greater emphasis is given to finding the common ground, enlarging the pie, generating alternatives that satisfy both parties, and looking for integrative solutions to problems (Pruitt 1983).

Finally, and perhaps most important, management stability provided trust. As discussed further in Chapter 7, trust is based on fulfilling the mutual expectations that each party has of the other. To define these mutual expectations requires time—to exchange information, to clarify roles and responsibilities, to test the relationship, and to observe results. Stability of the top management team provided the opportunity for trusting relationships to develop. Interpersonal capital could be accumulated over time, which could be drawn on in difficult situations. In contrast, institutions that lacked such stability had less capital to draw on in times of stress. The chief operating officer from one institution that had experienced considerable CEO turnover over the years explained the problem as follows:

> The current CEO has only been here a year longer than I have. And it takes some time before they get to know who you are, and there's been some turnover here in administration. I think there's a feeling now that the board is backing this administration and that there isn't going to be quick turnover. So in addition to the trust and credibility that comes from that, I think they know we're here for a while. When I first came here, I used to get comments about "You know, you guys come for two, three years and you're gone. We're here forever. The track record hasn't been all that good. And

we sit here holding the bag after you walk off to your next job." We got a lot of that at first, and we have to overcome that history.

The findings pertaining to management stability are particularly salient given the growing turnover of CEOs in the hospital industry (American College of Healthcare Executives and Heidrick and Struggles 1988). The unrest caused by turnover has profound effects on hospital-physician relationships. During the course of the study, one institution lost its highly respected CEO, and the anxiety is reflected in the following physician's comments: "We have real concern about who the new person is going to be. We trusted [previous CEO] so much. We've made a lot of progress, but now all of that could be threatened." These situations require strong board and medical staff leadership to help guide the institution during the period of transition.

Management Style: Leadership and Decision Making

As American productivity has fallen and foreign competition increased, there has been renewed interest in the topic of leadership and executive decision making (Burns 1979; Bass 1985; Garfield 1986; Bennis and Nanus 1985; Burns and Becker 1988; Kouzes and Posner 1988). The essence of management is in making choices among alternatives associated with achieving meaningful goals (McDaniel 1985). Each executive has a philosophy about how best to exercise influence and "make things happen." Managerial style or the formal leadership exercised by the CEOs in the present study played an important and pervasive role in promoting effective relationships. While not a sufficient condition, it was clearly a necessary condition for promoting and maintaining such relationships. Among the elements that stood out were

1. the manager's personal attitude toward physicians
2. their overriding commitment to open, honest communication
3. their use of overarching goals to build commitment and develop common ground
4. their resistance to overmanaging, thereby developing those under them to take on more responsibility
5. the way in which they involved physicians in decision making

Personal Attitude toward Physicians.   Almost without exception, the CEOs in the study sites genuinely liked and respected physicians. In fact, the opportunity to work with physicians, nurses, and other health care professionals is what attracted many of these individuals to the field. They treated physicians as individuals, appreciated their professional career objectives, and understood the many economic, regulatory, and legal pressures on their practices. They did not see physicians as the enemy. They recognized that each physician was different, and they understood and appreciated the multiple dimensions of physician roles—as the patient's agent, as a professional artisan, as an applied scientist, as a small business person, and as an entrepreneur. Depending on the given issue, they recognized that physician interests could be competitive or collaborative. When conflicts arose, they did not personalize them but rather attempted to understand them from the physician's perspective. As a result, they attempted to broaden the options that might meet both parties' needs. Recognizing that they had to live with physicians for the long run, they did not hang on to grudges associated with temporary disagreements. In brief, these CEOs had an ability to empathize; they were good "bridgers." At the same time, they had an ability to communicate the hospital's position. They did not kowtow to physicians. They could say no forcefully and persuasively in a manner that increased physician respect for administration rather than having it diminished. They asked for and largely received the same amount of respect, understanding, and trust that physicians demanded of administration. The following accounts bring these points to life.

> Our [CEO] likes doctors. He doesn't feel inferior and defensive around doctors. He genuinely respects their gifts, and he genuinely respects their talent. It is my belief that a lot of people who aren't physicians but have to work with physicians tend to underestimate them because they [physicians] frequently won't talk very much about things. They are either silent or make radical, passionate, irrelevant pronouncements and give the impression as being kind of lightweights in the management arena. This is frequently the impression nonphysicians have of physicians, and they get burned from time to time because physicians turn out to be much more perceptive than they thought. Our CEO really never underestimates physicians. He never underestimates their perception. And it's hard to hide the truth from intelligent people of all types. People who we deal with always read us better than we think they're doing. And that's in the area where [the CEO] is very, very good. So he doesn't need to beat up on physicians and show physicians he's better than them. He has a real affection for physicians. I think that's a very important aspect of our success.

Another executive states his views as follows:

> I think you start by liking physicians. I mean I like doctors, and I'd like to instill that mentality at the corporate level. We start with the

premise that there's this fundamental identification with physicians as people. I think there's a respect for not only the importance of physicians in terms of their contribution to your institutional success, but in terms of what they do, the contribution they make, and not just to your institution but to the community. I think if you don't have that respect, if you find an environment of distrust and dislike, then you find physicians are able to see through this pretty quickly. You can talk all you want about the bonding of physicians in the hospital, but unless there's this fundamental respect you have a credibility problem.

. . . I'd like to believe that they also feel we bring a professional competence and that they respect us for that. Not only do you have a higher purpose, but you can bring a capability to achieve that purpose through good management and good professional skills. And I think that when you roll it all together, they tend to sort of relate to you.

. . . I don't think it's a question of having to agree on every issue. Once I had a physician friend of mine who commented about an administrator: "Boy, we don't always agree and we'll arm wrestle sometimes on issues, but nothing is ever done under the table. I mean we know where we stand, and that's important. So we're willing to live with some differences, as long as we all have an understanding of where things are going and what the issues are that we're dealing with." You know, frankly, I think that's a pretty high testimony. We don't always live up to that, but I think if physicians get to the point that they don't quite know what your agenda is and they don't quite believe you are sharing what's important and what they need to know, then credibility and trust are eroded. And it's the old saying—if you get a crack in the glass, all they see is the crack. So you have to really avoid getting that crack in the glass.

An executive at another study site commented:

By example and by preaching, I've tried to instill our senior management team with the idea that physicians are our friends, our allies. Although some of my colleagues would say it's an outmoded concept, I think the essence of the role of the hospital executive is to facilitate the practice of medicine. Today, that's not just in inpatient settings. It covers the continuum of care. If you really operationalize that little piece of homespun philosophy, it markedly shapes how you deal with your medical staff.

An example of how to say no and still maintain respect is illustrated by the following hospital board member's comments:

> We had a situation where some physicians wanted more money, and the hospital had previously just provided them with more money time after time. Finally, [the new CEO] just laid down the law and said: "Look, this is how much we've been giving you, and we're not going to give you anymore." I think they respected him for it. Just like any time when you're in that type of situation, you usually end up attaining respect because the people knew they were basically doing wrong. In another instance I recall a physician who was causing a lot of problems with the hospital, and [the CEO] just asked him if he would please take his patients to another facility. He was harassing the nurses sexually and trying to get the hospital into lawsuits. He was not a nice person!

Still another CEO notes:

> I genuinely like physicians, and I've worked to develop a management team that feels the same way. I cleaned house when I took over because we had some who seemed to resent physicians and were openly hostile. We don't want that. I don't want my staff bad-mouthing physicians whether in public or behind their backs. That's not the atmosphere we create here.

Open, Honest Communication. A passionate, almost single-minded, commitment to open, honest communication was the one characteristic that stood out among nearly all CEOs. This was the sine qua non for developing and maintaining trust and credibility. Respondents emphasized the importance of bringing problems out in the open, of striving for accuracy in communication, of admitting mistakes, of not promising too much, of explaining the context in which the decision would be made, and of emphasizing the importance of follow-up and follow-through. The vice president for nursing at one of the institutions illustrates the point:

> I make rounds throughout the hospital to be on the floors where the physicians are and to know what's going on. You can have a casual conversation and a lot of times you can accomplish a lot more that way than through a formal committee meeting. The administrator and the assistant administrator both make the time to go to physicians' offices and ask, what's going on, what do you need, and where do you want to go with your practice?

The CEO at the same institution notes:

> Having the doctors come to me and talk about what's happened over the last four years has helped. We've tried to be responsive to their problems and eliminate obstacles. Having open and honest communication with doctors and not lying to them or trying to bluff them is important. And in today's health care arena, that's particularly important given all of the game playing going on.
>
> It's also important to understand historical events. In listening to doctors you have to realize that they also have hidden agendas. If you don't understand the historical events that preceded you, what may sound like a fantastic idea and a good suggestion may be made because the doctor has an agenda of why he wants it accomplished. And it may not necessarily be because of patient care. It may be because that he's got some little side war going on with another doctor, and this may be a one-upmanship type of thing. And I see that happen routinely where there are all of these side events going on. A lot of doctors feel that they're such astute businessmen and they get involved in these ludicrous financial deals, and they get p.o.'d at a doc because they feel he's reneged on a financial obligation, or he got involved in a situation and is losing money. So he uses the hospital infrastructure many times for his own political agenda. And you've got to ferret these out and address them openly.

The chief of staff at another institution noted:

> In general, administration has been open and honest. But they sometimes make mistakes in being overly certain of their own abilities. They make up plans without adequate physician input and then are surprised when physicians don't respond immediately. But, on the other hand, each time they do that, they've come out and admitted their mistake and backed off. Overall, they've been responsive to physician needs.

Additional communication issues are highlighted in Chapter 6.

Using Overarching Goals. Overarching goals are those that appeal to divergent interests in helping to create a shared vision. Given the divergent backgrounds and interests of hospitals and physicians, as discussed in Chapter 1, a particularly challenging aspect of the relationship is the search for common ground. In the sites studied, CEOs were adept at finding goals and causes that many, if not all, physicians could relate to both intellectually (that is, consistent with their ideals) and behaviorally (that is, important to their economic well-being and professional objectives).

The first step was the need to get to know their physicians, learn their needs, desires, and aspirations. This required time and the ability to listen. Surveys of physician offices helped, but often more mileage was gained from personal visits made by executives to physician offices and one-on-one meetings over breakfast, lunch, or dinner.

Once physician needs, aspirations, and desires were identified, the next step was to compare these with the hospital's mission and strategic plan, looking for or creating areas of overlap. Often, outside competition and cost-containment pressures were used to underscore the interdependency of the two groups and their mutuality of interest.

Once areas of overlap and mutual interest were identified, they had to be communicated to physicians and others in a way that moved them to action. CEOs used both their personalities and the office to imbue the overarching goal with symbolic power that would grab people emotionally. Most often, the overarching goals involved appeals to quality, maintaining professional responsibility, and autonomy.

By developing a set of overarching goals that both physicians and hospitals could buy into, many of the study sites were able to anticipate changes that might threaten their goals. This sometimes led to an ability to address issues before they became major problems or, in effect, to change before one really needed to change, as reflected in the comments of a McAuley physician:

> We have a philosophy here of excellence, of service, and of looking ahead. I have great respect for the medical center's forward planning and that includes the medical staff leadership who are brought along by the expertise of the marketers and businesspeople and administration. I would say that the administration has been more visionary than has the medical staff, but, relatively, this medical staff is quite conversant with the problems that are with us now and the problems yet to come. They have been made aware of these problems. Things were coming down the pipe, and steps were taken five and ten years ago to position the institution. . . . For example, the satellite program was underway early on. I think the effort at a joint venture HMO was ahead of its time. We didn't have to do that. We had such a controlled market area in Ann Arbor. We're living in candy land. So they really didn't have to do all of those things as early as they were done, but they did them I think in a very timely fashion. Of course, there was a lot of inertia

on the part of the medical staff to leave things as they were. Everybody was happy, making a good living, and the nature of the beast is not to make disruptive changes and certainly not to shake hands and get in bed with hospital administration. . . . The administration embraced the leadership of the medical staff, and the medical staff was responsive. I can think of maybe ten or maybe even fifteen years ago the preliminary and almost adolescent efforts that were made in undertaking strategic planning. I said this is ridiculous, but it turned out to be very worthwhile.

Resistance to Overmanaging.   When the environment becomes more stressful and problems more complex, the natural tendency is to try and exert greater personal managerial control. This, of course, usually makes the situation worse both because tighter control inhibits the creativity required for innovative solutions to difficult problems and because no single person (that is, the manager exerting greater control) has all the required abilities, knowledge, or experience to deal with complex events. Instead, what is needed in such times is not an increase in managerial control, but an increase in managerial competence and diversity. Rather than dealing with managerial control as a zero-sum game ("I have it and you don't"), one needs to expand the managerial competence and responsibility of everyone associated with the organization. This requires resisting the natural tendency to exert more control and having the courage to let go. It involves focusing one's time and energy on developing colleagues and subordinates. This "manager as developer" style (Bradford and Cohen 1984) was a key factor in the success of several of the CEOs studied. The following examples are illustrative. The first involves a board member at one of the institutions describing its CEO:

> He is a very complex person. He does not overmanage, he allows people to make mistakes, and this includes department heads and the hospital staff. He's not looking over someone's shoulder trying to figure out what they're doing wrong or correcting them with every little mistake that they make. He lets people make mistakes and learn from the mistakes similar to the way that a good parent would do. You just let your child experience things and find out what's right and what's wrong and make mistakes. And I think that's very difficult for a manager to do because I think a lot of people get into management and they want to control. They like the power, the ego, and all that, and [CEO] is not like that at all.

An executive at a second institution comments about his CEO as follows:

> I think [name of CEO] is a different kind of leader than a lot of them I've heard about or been exposed to. I call him kind of a gut reactor. And that works really well for him. It wouldn't for a lot of people, but he seems to have some intuitiveness about him and he's savvy enough that he knows all the little parts that are being played. He's able to make decisions fairly rapidly without a lot of formal analysis. I think he goes through it mentally in his head roughly. But he doesn't need a whole operations plan in front of him. He doesn't need to see every dollar and cent. He just has the sense for it. And I think he conveys that down through his administrative staff. He's very open to letting you try things. You know, if you want to try it, if it works—fine. If it doesn't work, then it doesn't work. But kind of one of the nice things about working here is that he allows you to be ingenious and come up with your own new ideas, and he'll encourage you to do that. You know, you don't even necessarily have to pass them by him. If it's in your area and it looks like it will work—just try it.

Involving Physicians.   Because they liked physicians, believed in open, honest communication, used overarching goals to build common ground, and believed in expanding the overall managerial competence of the organization, the CEOs of the study sites saw physician involvement as critical to their institution's success. While a number of factors influenced the type and staging of involvement, nearly all encouraged a participative process and support of greater physician involvement in the organization. As a physician executive at Sutter commented:

> Dealing with physicians is not always the easiest thing in the world. They are all individual entrepreneurs, and that's what they are raised to be. They are independent and difficult to deal with. But the CEO has always had an open door policy. Even to this day, doctors that are discontented with anything have free access to him. He'll bump it all to me or to [another executive] to take care of, but they have access to him and they know it. He comes routinely to medical staff meetings and is there to control rumors. During that time he'll address the issues that he knows are out there and answer questions that come up from the floor. You know, the best way to solve a problem is to hit it head on and get it out in the open. That just seems to be his modus operandi, and it seems to be working.

Another executive illustrated his participative style in handling capital expenditure requests as follows:

> We had budgeted $1.3 million and they [the physicians] came in at $2.0 million. I got them together and I said, "I've got this dilemma. You've requested $2 million of equipment, I can defend all of it, but here's the limitation." And I said, "You know, I'm going to ask you to do something I've never done before, but I think it will work. I want you to take time over the next 48 hours as a group to look at all this and prioritize it for me, instead of having hospital management do it." And they did and it worked out just fine.

Respondents also shared some of the complexities of the involvement process. As described by one CEO:

> In the early 1980s, we determined that we needed to have more geographic dispersion in the metropolitan area. One way to do that was to open the area's first urgent care center. We even targeted an area in the community where there were no particular loyalists. It was an area way out in the suburbs that, according to the health system's agency, was underserved. It also offered a lower cost alternative to our emergency rooms, so we had a lot of good reasons to get into it. Everybody bought off on that including the medical staff executive committee, and we felt we had done all the right things. In fact, we held a little wine and cheese tasting out there for community physicians to explain to them what we were going to do, and how they would benefit from all of the referrals of the urgent care center. But when we opened it, bearing in mind that this was the first one, all hell broke loose. It became a cause célèbre of the medical society. One primary care physician out there actually succeeded in getting his picture in the local paper about this giant hospital forcing him out of practice. I couldn't believe the photograph. He was sitting in a high-backed easy chair with a pipe and a dog at his knee. I mean it was unbelievable. It was just, you know, out of Norman Rockwell, and there was a big uproar that lasted for weeks. If it hadn't been for the fact the medical executive committee and board had been specifically involved in the process, I probably would have been fired. What came out of that was that the medical executive committee went to bat for this strategy. They said to their colleagues who were raising hell all over town: "Hey, we knew what was going to happen and we understand why the hospital did it, so shut up." I was really proud of them. At their next meeting, they admitted that maybe they were the best communications conduit to the staff at large.

The importance of involvement in making better decisions is also indicated by the following comment:

> The hospital is sometimes accused of taking forever to make a decision. I think decisions could be made more promptly, but I would rather have a good decision than a prompt bad one. But, I think we could do better. I think if we tend to err we do it on the side of too many committee meetings, too much time, too much agonizing, but I think that is kind of the style. [The CEO] would much rather err on that side than he would on making some snap judgment that turns out to be wrong. And you can see right on down through the administrative staff that his attitude and style permeates the whole atmosphere. His style is friendly, involving, persuasive, knowledgeable, tough when he needs to be, and caring. He is a pretty unique guy.

Physician Leadership

Involvement is a two-way process. Most of the study sites were fortunate in having strong physician leadership willing and able to accept responsibility. Such leadership stemmed from many sources. Some of it grew from a history of involvement and nurturing. This resulted in a sense of responsibility to keep the leadership strong. As expressed by a West Allis physician: "We have had an unbroken string of good chiefs of staff. No one wants to screw it up."

In other cases, management worked hard over a period of many years to develop staff leadership. As expressed by a Scripps physician: "I think the maturation of physician organizational skills is very important. I think that takes time. For us, I think it has taken fully ten years, and I don't think we're there yet. I think in another couple of years we will be there. I don't think it can happen quickly even when you have a number of responsible and sophisticated people as we do."

Many of the sites engaged in active programs of physician management development. These included participation in conferences, institutes, and seminars; university-based management courses; extending the terms of office for physician leaders; creating five nonvoting positions on the medical staff executive committee to expose young physicians to hospitalwide issues; rehearsing meetings with the medical staff executive committee; pushing decisions back down to the departments as appropriate; and generally reinforcing and encouraging medical staff responsibility for decision making. As expressed by a West Allis board member: "We try to see their [the doctors'] problems from the doctors' perspective. We try to be absolutely honest with them and we try to make them [the medical staff leadership] effective."

The effectiveness of physician leadership at Lexington is evidenced by their approach to communication. As one staff leader noted: "We have open forum meetings twice a year to make sure that we are getting across to the staff at large. We ask them: 'Are you hearing enough? Do you have any questions?'"

Having a medical director also played a positive role in several sites. The medical director was able to represent physicians' interests and views both within the hospital and externally to outside groups; facilitate and clarify communication between physicians and administration and reinforce feedback communication from administration to physicians; and sense and anticipate developing issues and unrest. Several CEOs used their medical director as a key confidant and as a sounding board for developing ideas and new strategic thrusts. In addition to a paid medical director, approximately half the sites compensated the chief of staff and some other physicians for time spent in administrative responsibilities.

Still another factor was the role played by physician groups. At least two sites, Sutter and Tucson Medical Center, had a number of physicians organized into group practices. As expressed by one Tucson physician:

> We organized into small groups, mostly single specialty. We also have a couple of multispecialty groups. There is usually one person in each office who can serve as a communicator back to the group. . . . This has helped with the decision-making process. This helps the communication problems in that you're not dealing with individual doctors, you're dealing with two groups. At least one person out of the group can become informed and educate the rest of the group. They start to indoctrinate each other to group action in contrast to the old individual approach.

It is also important to note that the medical staff leadership extends beyond the executive committee to other processes throughout the institution. In regard to capital expenditures, a Sutter physician noted:

> We have a committee of medical staff people that go through and talk to the department heads to see how much equipment is needed. We meet and argue as to who gets the first priority. It is a very interesting process. And, generally, we end up reducing a budget request that starts out at about six million down to about two million. It is amazing how the committee has matured and has developed a very statesmanlike approach to those things.

The effects of having strong physicians are evidenced at Providence Medical Center, where an executive commented:

> With very strong physician leadership we are able to work with the primary care physicians to get the consensus from key people to help build support for our primary care clinics. I am sure that the success of the project would not have occurred without the participative approach that we did in planning with them. There is lots of physician involvement. . . . I suppose underneath it, too, there is this sense of mutual respect in terms of openness between the administration and the medical staff. . . . It would be much more difficult for me today to accomplish some of these things than it was when we accomplished them at that time.

Examples of the importance of physician leadership extend beyond the study sites. At Santa Rosa Medical Center in San Antonio, Texas, a campaign was recently launched to delegate authority as close as possible to patient care activities and recruit physicians for participation in the hospital strategic planning process. The administration asked physicians to provide leadership in the formation of a new regional cancer program. As noted by Alex White, the hospital CEO: "We asked Dr. Parmiley for his leadership and he responded. The entire regionalization project is a microcosm of a program approach we intend to use again and again." (Health Care Productivity Report 1989, 5).

Evidence of physician leadership at Queen of the Valley Hospital in Napa, California, is reflected in the medical staff developing its own mission statement, shown in Exhibit 5.1.

CONTINGENCIES AFFECTING DECISION INVOLVEMENT

The decision-making process is complex. Too often the complexities are glossed over. Guidelines or suggestions are developed, which at first glance appear to hold true across a variety of conditions and circumstances, but which, in fact, break down in their implementation as a result of a number of contingencies and contextual circumstances that surround the decision-making process. Among these contingencies are the nature of the decision (strategic versus operational), the complexity of the decision, the importance of the decision, the stage of the decision-making process, and characteristics of the participants involved. Each of these affect the forms of involvement.

Exhibit 5.1   Mission Statement of the Medical Staff of Queen of the
                  Valley Hospital, Napa, California

A COMMITMENT TO VALUES
Medical Staff, Queen of the Valley Hospital

We have committed to being leaders in shaping our society's health care. We believe that we must serve the broad health needs of persons: spiritual, physicial,
social, and emotional.

We stand at the heart of the health care services, interacting with patients,
families, professional colleagues, agencies and institutions. As medical staff
members of the Queen of the Valley hospital, we are associated with an institution
which has a strong tradition of values. We are vital partners in the concrete ex-
pression of those values. Therefore, we offer the following statement.

We believe:

Life is sacred. We should courageously defend life but should not do so
when all attempts to preserve life are futile.

Sickness and healing are important events that effect all dimensions of a person's life. Physicians should address the spiritual, emotional and social dimensions of illness.

Informed competent patients are their own primary decision makers. Our
decisions about patient care involve the professional expertise and the personal
values of the patient, family and professionals. The conscience of the physicians
should be respected by patients and institutions.

Quality patient care is effected by clear, respectful, communication between
family and health care professionals.

Nurses have a unique relationship with doctors, patients, and the patient's
families. Their presence and expertise is of great importance in the care of patients.

Human dignity demands that our society insure universal access to an adequate level of health care. Physicians should play an active role in this process.

Physicians should serve on medical staff and peer review committees. Physicians should constructively challenge the goals of the institution and examine
with insight their own role and level of performance.

Only a community of shared vision can achieve these far reaching goals. We commit ourselves to be part of a community to work for these goals. We recognize that
resources are limited and require hard choices. We will join in making such
choices as fairly and accountably as possible.

Reprinted with the permission of Queen of the Valley Hospital.

Strategic versus Operational Decisions

Strategic decisions are those that position the organization relative to the environment and competition. They typically involve the core mission of the institution and its underlying values and assumptions. Operational decisions are those associated with implementation of the strategic plans and initiatives. They are concerned with who will do what, when, and how. Studies of other professional groups suggest that their main interest is in operational autonomy, not strategic autonomy (Bailyn 1985). In fact, if anything, they desire strategic direction from management. Health care may be different, however, in the need to involve at least some physicians in setting the overall strategic direction of the institution because of the close association that exists between strategic and operational issues.

While physicians are typically involved in operational decisions that affect them, recent research suggests that they are not involved in the important strategic decisions facing the institution (McDaniel 1990). This is particularly true in competitive markets (Alexander, Morrisey, and Shortell 1986) and for hospitals attempting to differentiate themselves from competitors based on quality-of-service criteria as opposed to cost criteria.

A distinguishing characteristic of many of the hospitals studied was their attempt to involve physicians more heavily in the strategic decisions. Nine out of ten hospitals studied, for example, had a relatively formal strategic planning process with committees composed of at least one-third physicians. While the tenth institution did not have a formal strategic planning process, strategic planning was done by administration and the hospital board, composed of five physicians.

While recognizing the importance of physician involvement in strategic planning in decision making, the hospitals experienced three major problems. The first was that often physicians were not involved early enough in the process. Although various issues might eventually be discussed at a retreat or within a strategic planning committee, physicians often perceived that the agenda and the underlying assumptions had already been determined by management, the board, or both. This is reflected in the following comments of a Sutter physician:

> I think there are some things that the hospital gets out ahead on. For instance, this new medical campus idea. I don't know if it was discussed very much by physicians. The idea that the hospital wanted to merge or acquire another hospital is another example. There wasn't much physician input into that proposal. Now maybe there was—I'm just not aware of it—but it was never anything that I was involved in as the chief of the department at the time. In

those major decisions, the administration tends to go by itself, whereas in some of the lesser decisions, such as where we should put a new radiology unit or ambulatory surgery facility, we get involved. I think in those areas the hospital tries to work with physicians. But in the big scheme, I think they tend to go their own way.

A Providence physician noted:

We often do too much processing. I've said this about 15 times. But what happens at a meeting is that it's all one-way communication. Management will tell us what they've been doing and how they see things going and what the solutions are going to be, and then they'll say, here's how you can help. This is not really participation at all. We recently had a presentation that was saying, here's the next five-year plan, and not one physician on the executive board had been consulted on it. In fact, we basically had to send them back to the drawing board because we felt their whole basic vision of how health care emanates was off-base.

A second problem involves keeping physicians continuously involved in the process. Several institutions made major time investments in launching strategic plans with heavy physician input, but they often did not involve them in the implementation process or continue their involvement in the ongoing strategic planning process of the institution. The initial "fix" began to wear off. As expressed by one CEO:

When we completed the planning, we had a hell of a lot of work in front of us. Office buildings, clinics, programs to build, parking efforts to launch. We also had to bring our cost down since they were the highest in town. . . . When we did all of that planning, there was a lot of participation. Then we launched into this implementation stuff that became a management focus, and we didn't keep the physicians as involved in that phase. It took, I would say, a couple of years. We were able to ride on it for a couple of years. I would say we have lost part of that sense of involvement in ownership and what is going on, and I think it is because of focusing on management issues and implementation more than planning. So I guess what we need to do is get back to some of the original planning mechanisms we had.

A third problem involved the separation between medical staff leadership and the staff at large. While most medical staff leaders felt appropriately involved in the strategic planning process, they were the first to admit that the results did not seem to filter down to others. As one nonleader physician stated: "Oh, there should be much more. I think they're missing an opportunity for a lot of help. They're not doing it."

Efforts were made, however, to deal with each of these issues. Many sites used retreats to address emerging physician concerns and "get things back on track." An executive at Tucson Medical Center stated:

> Physicians are heavily involved in the annual strategic planning retreat, and I think we bare our souls pretty much in that process. We do a critical assessment of competitors and where we think our strengths and weaknesses are. We outline where we think some of the priorities are for the coming year. And the way which [the physician vice president for strategic planning] has organized natural breakout sessions in which just physicians talk to each other. Then we have mixed sessions in which the board, physicians, and management deal with issues. So the physicians' input in creating the future vision, I think, comes through very, very well.

As one executive at McAuley stated:

> They [the physicians] have had input into our shift in the role statement particularly as it relates to looking at our service areas and the expansion of those areas. They participated in that. We have had a lot of participation in helping to decide the number of physicians we're going to need and how we're going to recruit those physicians. Physicians are also heavily involved in each of our service line business plans that are being developed and that are driven by the overall strategic plan. They've been involved in developing and reacting to the goal statements, and as a result, we've added a specific goal that had to do with physician relations. This goal specified that physicians would have greater opportunities to influence events and to be recognized and rewarded.

Overall, the institutions were working to develop models of integrated, rather than fractionated, hospital-physician strategic planning (Kovner and Chin 1985). But, for the most part, the integration was limited to the physician leadership level and had not yet permeated many of the staff physicians at large. While it is unrealistic (and unnecessary) to expect the majority of physicians to undertake significant leadership responsibilities, no longer can physicians practice medicine unencumbered by managerial and organizational considerations, commitments, and responsibilities. It was in regard to the latter that a number of physician leaders expressed their frustrations with some of their colleagues.

Decision Complexity and Importance

Physician involvement is also affected by the complexity and importance of the decision to the institution. In general, the more complex and important a decision, the greater the need for early, persistent, and pervasive physician involvement. This involvement, however, cannot take place in an ad hoc fashion. Rather, the mechanisms or forums for such involvement must already be in place so energy can be focused rapidly on the evolving issues. This did not rule out the creation of ad hoc task forces. But these task forces had to be used appropriately and efficiently, with the right people involved, clear expectations of the charge, a common information base (Gill and Delbecq 1985), group meeting skills, and relevant professional leadership (Altier 1986). Most importantly, the task forces needed to be held accountable and linked to existing decision-making groups such as the medical staff executive committee, the department chairman's committee, or the strategic planning committee. (The negative effect of not following these guidelines is highlighted in the minicases at the end of this chapter). Those institutions with medical directors appeared to be better able to use task forces productively as the medical director played a key coordinative role in linking task force recommendations to appropriate decision-making bodies.

Examples of more complex important decisions that were associated with greater physician involvement included expanding primary care services, physician recruitment, development of joint ventures, discussion of a possible merger, initiatives to improve the institution's quality of care, and issues involving the implications of nurse shortages for nurse staffing. The following comments of a Tucson executive reflect his philosophy regarding nursing issues:

> I think we've got a good balance of physician involvement. Physicians aren't heavily involved in management from a day-to-day perspective. We offer them the opportunity to comment. For example, when we're filling a position of a nursing unit manager, we'll ask physicians who practice on that unit to be part of an interview team to provide input. They don't have the final vote, but we look to them to be involved. When I interviewed candidates for the nursing administrator position, I invited 18 physicians to be part of an interview group and had them spend two hours with each of the candidates. I asked for their feedback and then had separate meetings between the chief of staff and the candidates. So we look for their involvement, but we don't look to them to manage.

Sometimes, however, time does not permit extended involvement. In these cases, one needs to rely on trust that has been established through past involvement. As a Leonard Morse executive commented:

> You need enough marbles on your side to get away with a few quick decisions. You can do it if you've built up trust . . . as long as you go back to them and close the loop.

Decision-Making Stages

Five stages of the decision making process were identified:

1. raising the issue or identifying the problems
2. clarifying the problems
3. generating alternatives
4. evaluating alternatives
5. choosing the best perceived alternative

Physicians were not necessarily involved in the same way or to the same degree at each stage of the process. To a great extent, this depended on the nature of the problem as discussed above (that is, strategic versus operational, complexity, and importance).

Physicians were particularly helpful in the early stages of issue identification and problem clarification. Several executives noted that without physician participation in these stages, the clinical significance and implications of plans would have been missed. These included decisions involving outpatient treatment for AIDS, the development of an outpatient mental health unit, and expansion of a hospital's rehabilitation unit. As medicine becomes more complex and new technologies continue to evolve, clinical input into the early stages of the process will grow. Most sites saw this as one of the major reasons to involve physicians in the strategic planning and decision-making processes of the institution at all levels.

Physician input was frequently found useful in generating and evaluating alternatives as well. Their input at these stages, however, was largely from the clinical perspective and, perhaps, more narrowly from a specific subspecialty perspective. Such input needs to be balanced with other perspectives. For example, in attempting to solve a problem of a shortage of intensive care unit nurses, a Tucson executive noted:

> I brought the physicians together and said: "One of the problems is you want quality patient care for your patients, but in order to

respond to that I'm having to bring in agency nurses. From my perspective, they aren't committed to the philosophy of the institution. They are just here to make a buck. And I don't think your patients in the long run are going to benefit. Now there are things I have to do to get some issues resolved, but there are some things you all need to do for us too, including the way you write orders. If you require one-to-one nursing, we need more nurses. You need to be more sensitive to the implications that has for staffing and our ability to respond. You need to pay attention to your attitude and how you relate to nurses. If you don't create an attractive environment, I can't hire the nurses because they won't want to work with you. You have a responsibility to be more collegial. And also at some point in time, if I have too many agency staff, I do think there's a safety issue. I want you to know that I'm going to divert patients and if we need to, we'll close down the emergency room."

The final stage of making a choice was seldom made by physicians alone, but rather by management after considerable physician input into the earlier stages. For the most part, physicians did not expect to be the final decision makers but very much wanted the opportunity to influence the process, to be listened to, and to see their ideas and suggestions taken seriously.

A related key to success was involving physicians at the right time. The opportunity cost of most physicians' time is very high. Therefore, their involvement must be carefully structured to maximize the benefit for both the hospital and the physician. The issue of timing is illustrated by the situation at one hospital, which faced a drug bust involving several employees in the hospital's radiology department. As the hospital's executive noted:

This drug bust could have gone one way or the other. This was an example of working together with the medical staff. They were so appreciative that we brought them in just at the right moment. They were fully briefed before the press got all over us, and they completely understood what we were doing. They became supportive as opposed to being in the dark and having to see it on TV.

Participant Characteristics

The form and effectiveness of physician involvement also depends on the characteristics of the participants themselves (Moore and Simendinger 1986). These include such characteristics as specialty, age, experience, form of practice, hospital loyalty, and, perhaps most importantly, an understanding of each physician's practice needs or "value chain" (Sheldon 1986, 110; Snook 1984). One participating CEO commented:

> I can pretty accurately categorize my medical staff. There are the rabble rousers who will oppose almost anything we do on principle. There are those who are pretty apathetic. They don't seem to care one way or the other. There are those who are supportive but are pretty traditional in their thinking and want to preserve things as much as possible. Then there are some hard chargers who want to do some new things; some entrepreneurs.

Depending on the issue, this CEO would involve different members of these four groups, in addition to the considerations of specialty mix, experience, and expertise relevant to the problem. Several CEOs emphasized the importance of involving some of the "nay-saying rabble rousers" in the decision-making process. In the words of one:

> We make it our policy to involve those who disagree with us. It has several advantages. It gives them the opportunity to be heard. They know we value their opinion even if we disagree. It also gives an opportunity to educate them and broaden their understanding of the hospital. And, perhaps most importantly, it forces us to reexamine our position in some of our assumptions. We never want people who only agree with us on our committees.

From the above, it is obvious that appropriate and effective physician involvement in decision making is a more subtle and complex process than merely counting the number of physicians on the board or strategic planning committee. It essentially involves a process of matching physician characteristics, skills, experiences, and needs with the nature of the decision to be made in terms of the strategic and operational complexity and importance of the decision and the stage of the decision-making process. It is important that the decision-making structure not be confused with the decision-making process, and that both be seen as relevant and supportive of hospital-physician interests.

As indicated above, there were many positive examples of appropriate and effective physician involvement in decision making. But the motivation to do so did not always come easily to the executives interviewed. As one commented:

> I frequently don't want them involved. I don't believe physicians are good managers at all, although there are some rare exceptions. You know their whole life has been one of independent operation where they make their own decisions and tell people what to do. They're not used to working as part of an organization where they

have to take directions sometimes. They're used to getting what they want. They look at things from a very narrow focus most of the time because they're directing what they need for their patient and they forget all of the other things.

As expected, the issue of involvement was usually more complex in institutions that were members of hospital systems. In these situations, physicians frequently felt a remoteness, and even fear of the corporate office, even though recent research suggests that systems are working hard to dispel such feelings (Burns, Andersen, and Shortell 1989). This occurred even where there existed a strong, trusting relationship with the local hospital CEO. Physicians feared that the corporate office would dictate policy, and that the local physicians would have little influence over things that might not be in their best interest. In particular, several were concerned that resources might be drained away from their hospital to support other more needy hospitals in the system. This was reflected in the comment of one physician:

The hospital here has made a commitment to putting [another hospital] up in [another part of the city]. They bought [still another site]. All of those things, I think, were economically motivated, survivor-oriented, and expansionistic. My honest, gut feeling is that there was zero physician input into any of those. Now, I'm not sure there should have been. I mean, as long as these guys are responsible about running a financially viable outfit, I don't care if they have 14 hospitals in [name of another state] as long as I can provide quality care here. But there wasn't any physician input into any of those decisions, and I think it might foster more trust and interaction between the medical staff and administration if they allowed such input. I will say that over the last year or two this seems to have changed. They're now more open about these things. But it's still like, we're telling you that we're thinking about it. It's not, hey, what do you think about this and should we do it?

The above statement underscores the initial discussion regarding the importance of early physician involvement, being able to question underlying assumptions and the structuring of the decision context versus being asked to provide input on strategic directions that are "already out of the shop."

MINICASE I

Most of the chapter has highlighted positive examples of managerial style and physician involvement. But even the best institutions make mistakes. A couple of examples are highlighted here. The first situation involves a planned joint undertaking between a group of cardiologists and the hospital to develop a stronger regional cardiology service. A task force jointly composed of hospital and cardiology program representatives was appointed to develop the expanded program. The cardiologists' goals, expectations, and time frame for implementation, however, turned out to be very different from those of the hospital. Neither party appeared to be sufficiently aware of this to take early corrective action. The situation began to unravel when the cardiology group hired its own marketing director, as it felt the program was nearing a launching point. Things finally exploded when a scheduled press conference announcing the formation of a new heart institute was canceled. In the words of an outside consultant:

> There are some very deep concerns about whether you [the cardiology group and the hospital] share the same values and goals and time frame. I don't know that any of you clarified these things from the time you started meeting until some things started happening. From what I can tell, there was never any specificity about exactly what the results of the investment, time, and energy would be.

In particular, the respective roles and responsibilities of the hospital vice president responsible for the cardiology service and the cardiology group's marketing director and program coordinator needed to be clarified. The latter individual was expected to serve two masters— the cardiology group and the hospital. The cardiology group felt that the individual was serving them exclusively. As a result, the decision context for both parties was very different. The hospital had many more stakeholders and constituents to consider in launching the new program than did the cardiologists. They did not appear to be aware of or appreciate the hospital's situation. At the same time, the hospital did not appear to appreciate or understand the physicians' desire to launch the new program as soon as possible, reflecting their concern with losing patients if a competitor developed a similar program more quickly. There was need for an overall game plan that included a clarification of roles, responsibilities, expectations, and time frames.

MINICASE II

At a second hospital, a situation developed in which the state workers' compensation carriers refused to pay bills. Hospital administration responded by attempting to force them to either pay their bills or not admit the patient. This created problems for the medical staff, who would call up the admitting office and learn that these patients were no longer being scheduled. The medical staff had not been informed of the hospital's decision. It was perceived by the medical staff as a "shoot from the hip" response. It ruffled a few feathers. It was eventually straightened out by the hospital explaining the situation. As one individual stated: "We have an administration that sometimes tends to shoot from the hip a little bit, and this is when we get in trouble. We have to keep reminding ourselves not to do this." The incident illustrates how a single event can threaten hard-earned trust. The situation called for direct communication with physicians in a timely fashion (see Chapter 6).

MANAGERIAL BEST PRACTICES ASSOCIATED WITH PHYSICIAN INVOLVEMENT

1. Physicians are strongly involved in the institution's overall strategic planning process. They typically make up at least a third of the membership of the strategic planning committee and are heavily involved in subcommittees, ad hoc task forces, reactor groups, and retreats.

2. Special efforts are made to involve younger physicians on the staff. They are targeted for involvement in key committees and participation in retreats. One hospital uses an administrator buddy system to work one-on-one with key younger physicians. Another hospital creates five nonvoting positions on the medical staff executive committee for younger physicians to help expand their horizons and orient them to medical staff leadership issues.

3. Special emphasis is placed on involving physicians throughout the institution and encouraging them to take responsibility for solving their own problems. The CEO and administration resist solving problems brought to them by the medical staff that should rightfully be handled by the staff and its executive committee. In turn, the medical staff executive committee does the same with the medical department heads and section chiefs. Considerable effort is made to solve problems at the lowest level of responsibility.

4. The CEO meets quarterly with the entire medical staff to discuss concerns and rumors. The CEO shares the rumors he or she has heard and openly discusses the elements of both fact and fiction.

5. Heavy use is made of retreats to educate, to expand horizons, to explore emerging problems, to reinforce the institution's culture, and to involve younger physicians.

6. Negative, complaining physicians are placed on committees considering important issues. "Don't just ask the people who agree with you."

7. A lot of discussion is held prior to key meetings in order to anticipate problems, air differences in advance, and extend the range of potential solutions. Often such meetings are held before the regularly scheduled medical staff executive committee meeting as a dry run. The meetings are used to anticipate issues and build a forum for managing conflict. They help to assure that no surprises occur.

8. A nurse-physician liaison committee is used to deal with issues arising out of the increased stress on both nurses and physicians.

9. Hospital board members are extensively involved in the hospital's quality assurance efforts. They are members of the quality assurance committee of the medical staff as well as the hospital and also serve on the credentials committee. Administration is also heavily involved in these activities. In some cases, the board has a medical policy committee that oversees the credentialing process. Annual written and verbal reports are made to this group by department chiefs.

10. The hospital uses a resource allocation/technology advisory committee composed primarily of physicians to prioritize requests for new equipment and technology.

11. A paid medical director/executive vice president for medical affairs is used to help facilitate strategic integration of different interests, promote effective two-way communication, assist the medical staff executive committee, and oversee more comprehensive and integrated quality assurance activities.

12. The hospital pays a stipend to the chief of staff and to other physician leaders who contribute a significant amount of time to managerial responsibilities.

REFERENCES

Alexander, J. A., M. A. Morrisey, and S. M. Shortell. 1986. "Effects of Competition, Regulation, and Corporatization on Hospital-Physician Relationship," *Journal of Health and Social Behavior* 27(September):220–35.

Altier, W. J. 1986. "Task Forces—An Effective Management Tool," *Sloan Management Review* (Spring):69–76.

American College of Healthcare Executives, American Hospital Association, and Heidrick and Struggles. 1988. *CEO Turnover Report*. Chicago: American Hospital Association.

Bailyn, L. 1985. "Autonomy in the Industrial R and D Lab," *Human Resource Management* 24(2):129–46.

Bass, B. M. 1985. *Leadership and Performance Beyond Expectations*. New York: The Free Press.

Bennis, W., and B. Nanus. 1985. *Leaders: The Strategies for Taking Charge*. New York: Harper and Row.

Bradford, D. L., and A. R. Cohen. 1984. *Managing For Excellence: The Guide to Developing High Performance in Contemporary Organizations*. New York: John Wiley and Sons.

Burns, J. W. 1979. *Leadership*. New York: Harper and Row.

Burns, L. R., R. M. Andersen, and S. M. Shortell. 1989. "The Impact of Corporate Structures on Physician Inclusion and Participation," *Medical Care* 27(10):967–82.

———. 1990. "The Effect of Hospital Control Strategies on Physician Satisfaction, Autonomy, and Hospital-Physician Conflict," *Health Services Research (in press)*.

Burns, L. R., and S. W. Becker. 1988. "Leadership and Managership," in S. M. Shortell and A. D. Kaluzny (Eds.), *Health Care Management: A Text in Organization Theory and Behavior*. 2nd ed. New York: John Wiley and Sons.

Garfield, C. 1986. *Peak Performers: The New Heroes of American Business*. New York: Morrow and Co.

Gill, S. L., and A. L. Delbecq. 1985. "Justice As a Prelude to Teamwork in Medical Centers," *Healthcare Management Review* 10(Winter):45–53.

Health Care Productivity Report, October 1989, 2, 11.

Kouzes, J. M., and B. Z. Posner. 1988. *The Leadership Challenge: How to Get Extraordinary Things Done in Organizations*. San Francisco: Jossey-Bass.

Kovner, A. R., and M. J. Chin. 1985. "Physician Leadership and Hospital Strategic Decision-Making," *Hospital and Health Services Administration* 30 (November/December):64–79.

Lang, D. 1988. *Medical Staff News* (November):3.

McDaniel, R. 1985. "Management and Medicine, Never the Twain Shall Meet," *Journal of the National Medical Association* 77(2):107–12.

———. 1990. "Patterns of Participation in Strategic Decision Making: The Case of Hospitals." Paper revised and resubmitted to *Organizational Science*.

Moore, T. E., and E. A. Simendinger. 1986. "How to Involve the Right Physicians in the Leadership Process," *Healthcare Forum* (May-June):61–66.

Pruitt, D. G. 1983. "Achieving Integrative Agreements," in M. J. Bazerman and R. J. Lewicki (Eds.), *Negotiating in Organizations*. Beverly Hills: Sage Publishers, 35–50.

Sheldon, A. 1986. *Managing Doctors*. Homewood, IL: Dow Jones–Irwin.

Snook, I. D., Jr. 1984. *Building a Winning Medical Staff*. Chicago, IL: American Hospital Publishing.

CHAPTER 6

Developing Effective Communication

Effective communication was one of the most frequently mentioned reasons for successful hospital-physician relationships. It was also mentioned as the most important contributor to the development of trust (see Chapter 7). Its importance is also documented by others (Georgopoulos, D'Aunno, and Saavedra 1987; Longest and Klingensmith 1988) and highlighted by the following comments of a McAuley physician:

> I think a lot of the staff have grown in their understanding of how important communication is in this environment. Neither one of us is going to come out on top if we don't communicate. . . . As the environment changes, it's harder. As money gets tighter, it's harder . . . but I do think we communicate well. I do think we involve physicians in decision making. They're on the board, they're on planning committees, they're on the strategic planning committee. They have all of these networks themselves. I think we've also had some well-chosen department heads.

While all agree on the importance of effective communication, there is a need to move beyond simple prescriptions and exhortations. This chapter develops a framework or model of communication that can be used by physicians and hospitals to improve their ability to communicate. Examples from the ten study sites are used to highlight key guidelines, and a set of communication best practices are identified.

A GUIDING FRAMEWORK

To be an effective communicator requires two things. First is the desire to communicate, and second is an understanding of how people learn.

In addition to one's personal values, the desire to communicate is influenced by the expectation that the communicative act or behavior will be rewarded or reinforced in a meaningful way. This may take several forms, but at the heart is the feeling that one has been listened to—that it was worth the time and effort involved. The other person doesn't necessarily have to agree with what was said or act on it, but they must provide us with some feedback indicating that they have heard what we said. As expressed by one physician respondent, "We have physicians and administrators using the same words but speaking a different language, and neither one of them knows it." One approach to ensure that a common language is being spoken and heard is to engage in "migrating." Migrating is the ability of a person hearing a message from another person to acknowledge in some way what the other person has said, whether or not one agrees with it (Neuhauser 1988). The ability to migrate is reflected in the following comments about a CEO at one of the study hospitals:

> I don't think I've seen a situation where people haven't felt heard. They may not agree at the end, or someone may be extremely belligerent, but they have felt listened to. He [the CEO] has a real strong sense of consensus, and he can really negotiate issues and get people to put their issues on the table. And, you know, sometimes that still results in less than total agreement, but at least people felt heard.

Understanding how people learn requires getting to know how they like to receive and process information. Some people prefer verbal communication, and others written communication. Some people learn best by observing other people's behavior, that is, actions speak louder than words. Some people are more analytical (that is, left brain–oriented), while others are more intuitive (that is, right brain–oriented). Those who are more analytical prefer lists of information, logical reasoning, the spelling out of assumptions, equations, and hard evidence. They want things wrapped up with conclusions drawn. Those who are more intuitive prefer anecdotes, stories, personal examples, and pictures. They do not require closure, prefer things open-ended, and like to see the possibilities in things.

While there are drawbacks to characterizing physicians only by their specialty, it does provide some clues to how they perceive and process information. Surgeons, for example, are more likely to be high on the analytical dimension and prefer things to be concrete. They relate better to communication that is presented in a logical, straightforward manner that includes concrete steps for action. Internists, while also analytical, will tend toward the abstract and intuitive. They tend to have a higher tolerance for ambiguity in communication than do surgeons. Internists are more willing to see the possibilities in what was not said as well as what was said. Family practitioners and pediatricians tend to communicate, and like to be communicated with, in people-oriented terms. They relate well to stories and messages that use people as examples and that have implications for people's behavior.

Thus, an effective communicator is a person who matches the form and method of communication to the preferences of the recipient. This is not easily done. Being open, honest, candid, and consistent is necessary but not sufficient. One needs to go beyond these prescriptions to become skillful at tailoring communication in a way that increases the probability that one will be heard—being willing to tailor messages to the needs and preferences of the would-be listeners, without compromising the "truth" of the message. This is somewhat easier to do in personal communication where one knows the other person, one of the reasons given by several CEOs for their frequent use of one-to-one communication with selected key physicians. This becomes more difficult, of course, when communicating with diverse groups (such as the medical staff at large), which have a variety of preferences regarding ways of learning. In these cases, the best advice is to pitch the message to the dominant orientation in the group (if there is one), use a variety of different approaches (for example, logical lists as well as pictures and stories) to get the message across, or both. There is also a need to reinforce what has been communicated in multiple ways—through one-on-one interaction, small group interaction, written memos, newsletters, video, and so on. Being an effective communicator requires considerable savvy and a lot of hard work.

In addition to the desire to communicate, and understanding how people learn, effective communication is also influenced by (1) the purpose of the message; (2) the content, importance, and complexity of the message; (3) the characteristics of the sender and receiver; and (4) the time frame under consideration. The purpose of the message may simply be to provide information, to elicit a response, or to arrive at a decision. One needs to consider whether the recipient of the message understands one's intent. This is a particular challenge when a new CEO has arrived or when a new chief of staff has taken office. People are used to understanding the intent and message of previous incumbents; they may require time and much clarification of messages in order to adjust to a new individual. For example, one CEO in the study expressed dismay when a discussion with the medical staff executive committee regarding the probability of sharing services with another hospital was perceived by the physicians present as a decision already made! This is because such messages from the previous CEO were, indeed, intended to communicate a decision that had already been made. The new CEO intended the message only as information for subsequent discussion (not even requiring a response at the present meeting) rather than as communicating a decision.

The preciseness of one's message—the cues that one uses to guide the likely response of the recipient—will vary as a function of its purpose. In general, one needs to be more precise as one moves from simply providing information, to attempting to elicit a response, to wanting to arrive at a decision. In providing information, the cue may be as general as: "This is all we currently know. We'll continue to keep everyone informed." In wanting to elicit a response, the cue must be somewhat more precise, along the lines of: "What is your reaction to this? What do we think about this? What additional information do we need?" If the intent is to arrive at a decision, there is a need to be quite precise in spelling out the underlying assumptions of the decision, the relevant alternatives, the pros and cons of each, the likely consequences, and the time frame of action. While these considerations may seem fundamental, they become more subtle when one remembers that they will be perceived differently by different kinds of physicians. Surgeons, for example, work on short time frames and are action oriented. They will, therefore, tend to overinterpret communication cues and may frequently interpret a message meant only to communicate information as a call for action. Pathologists and internists, on the other hand, may interpret a communication involving the need to make a decision as a call for still more information and analysis.

Providing feedback is a special aspect of communication. Such communication involves both providing information and eliciting a response. A number of suggestions growing out of the experiences of the study and existing literature (Athos and Gabarro 1978) are relevant:

1. The feedback should be given with attention. The communicator must be very aware of what is being said to the recipient and alert to the recipient's verbal and nonverbal responses.

2. The feedback should be directly expressed. Executives and physicians sometimes fall into communication traps due to the inclination to withhold information or make overly vague statements that are of little value. The most useful communication is direct, open, and concrete.

3. The feedback should be free of evaluative judgments. Situations and events should be described as you see them but should be done in a way that does not put the recipient on the defensive. If a judgment is offered, it should be clear that the issue is one of subjective evaluation. The other party should be invited to

make their own judgment and evaluation of the situation. In this fashion, engagement in joint problem solving can occur.

4. The feedback should be well timed. Feedback should be given when the receiver is receptive to it and should be sufficiently close to the event being discussed for it to be fresh in their mind. Storing up comments from the past can lead to a buildup of negative feelings and reduce the effectiveness of feedback when it is finally given.

5. Feedback should be readily actionable. It should center around behavior that can be changed by the receiver. Feedback concerning matters outside the control of the receiver is less useful. In addition, it is useful for those communicating feedback to suggest alternative ways of behaving that may allow the receiver to think about different ways of tackling the problems identified.

The content, importance, and complexity of the issue associated with the communication are also factors to consider. In the case of hospital-physician communication, the content may range from a physician-credentialing issue, to a joint venture, to a proposal for improving quality assurance. The message may involve various combinations of data, ideas, and examples. It may vary in importance and complexity. The more important and complex the issue, the greater the need to attend to the recipient's preferences for learning. Of course, hospitals and physicians do not always agree on the importance of given issues. For example, a controversial decision involving the renewal of a physician's privileges may be viewed as a much more important and symbolic decision by physicians than hospital administration, who sees it only as a single case among many. Conversely, the hospital's interest in improving productivity may be seen by hospital executives as central to long-run survival, while physicians may see it as only a tangential nuisance to established practice patterns and protocols. The situation, of course, is frequently much more complex than this since physician subgroups view different issues with varying degrees of importance.

Communication can be used to raise or lower the saliency of given issues by placing them in a larger context. For example, in the HMO and managed care case, study executives frequently raised the importance of these issues to physicians by pointing out the implications for physician practices and the threat of growing competition to physicians, in addition to the implications for the hospital. The message was tailored to the perceived needs and interests of different groups. For the specialists, the threat to referrals was emphasized. For the primary care physicians, the direct loss of patients to other physicians was highlighted.

Another common strategy used by study executives was bringing in outsiders to communicate the message. Outsiders often provided variety and additional credibility to the issue by offering concrete examples. The message often was "if it happened to us, it could happen to you, too." Or in a more positive vein: "We decided to take things into our own hands and have some control over our destiny, and you can too."

Complex, ambiguous issues offered particular challenges to effective communication. They required a "whole-parts-whole" communication framework. First, it is important to provide a description of the larger picture, the overall goal, and the context in which behavior and issues are likely to evolve. Next, it is important to break down the issue into manageable components, with a clear set of expectations regarding how each component will be addressed. Then, from time to time, it is necessary to return to the larger picture and show how the various subcomponents are related to each other and how they address the larger issues and goals involved.

Complex, ambiguous issues also require using a combination of lean and rich media (Daft and Lengel 1986). Lean media involves written communication and is useful for providing facts and figures that can help reduce uncertainty. Rich media involves face-to-face discussions individually and in groups and is required to move people to action. The most effective communication includes judicious use of both lean and rich media.

An example of the whole-parts-whole and lean vs. rich approaches was provided by one hospital's discussion of a proposed merger with another institution. Considerable attention was at first given to the broad picture, using primarily facts and figures and then moving to discussion of the consistency with the hospital's mission, values, and long-run objectives. The issues were then broken down into specific components, such as the compatibility of specific service offerings, managed care networks, and the strengths and weaknesses of the respective institutions. These were carried on in smaller groups. Periodically, they were related back to the bigger picture. The hospital is currently engaged in an ongoing back-and-forth process of communication and discussion involving multiple groups. In the process, they are attempting to balance the need for detail and closure with the need for openness, fluidity, and the sensing of multiple possibilities.

Considering the characteristics of the sender of the message and the recipient are important for effective communication. From the sender's perspective, the main issue is one of credibility. Credibility, of course, is linked with trust (as discussed in Chapter 7) and depends on both ascribed (for example, one's formal position, family background, and physical appearance) as well as achieved characteristics (for example, one's abilities, knowledge, skills, and accomplishments). An important lesson from the executives studied was that they seldom relied on or appealed to their ascribed characteristics or official positions to increase the credibility of their communication. Rather, their credibility as communicators was based on the trust developed between them and their physicians as a result of past experience: being open and honest, and doing what they said they were going to do. Further, they went to great lengths to expand the communication credibility of their management team so that communication from any member of the management team would be viewed as equally credible by physicians as communication directly from the CEO, as reflected in the comments of the following physician at North Monroe:

> They've all been very helpful. I work with [the vice president for nursing], and I also work with [the controller]. The two controllers before the present controller I got to know pretty well, and I really liked both of them as far as being easy to get in touch with and to talk to, and they've been very helpful. A lot of times if [the CEO] was busy you could talk to someone else, and they would relay the message adequately to where it was taken care of. It's probably not their job but when you can't get in touch with the administrator after rounds or something, you can just stop by and talk to one of them and they'll take care of it. All of them have been really good.

What this physician didn't realize is that it *was* their job and was a very important part of the CEO's management development philosophy.

Ascribed characteristics such as medical specialty can serve as a helpful shortcut for targeting messages. But, as in the case of the sender of the message, greater reliance was generally placed on the achieved experience of working with physicians and learning who could be trusted with certain kinds of information and who could not. Similarly, when physicians were the senders of communication and administration the recipients, the credibility of the message was largely evaluated based on the credibility of the sender as a function of past experience, rather than the individual's ascribed position. A particular challenge was communicating with those physicians who were not elected staff leaders, section heads, or committee heads.

Still another factor affecting communication is the time frame associated with the content of the communication. The shorter the time frame involved, the more precise the communication cues (see above) that need to be provided. More concrete examples, discussion of consequences, and calls for action need to be made a part of the message. Hearing the same message from several different people also helps.

Where the time frame involved is longer, communication cues can be more general, abstract, and open-ended.

The major factors associated with effective communication are shown in diagram form in Figure 6.1. The desire to communicate and understanding how others learn directly influence the probability of effective communication taking place. But, as shown, one also needs to take into account the purpose and content of the communication, the credibility of the sender, and the time frame involved. Increasing effective communication reinforces the desire to communicate in the future and, therefore, increases the level of trust between the parties involved. It is the fuel that drives the relationship.

SOME EXAMPLES FROM THE FRONT LINE

Learning to Say No

From an executive at Crouse-Irving Memorial:

> I think that communication is the best thing that I can put on the table in dealing with the medical staff. They're not easy to deal with. I think that you have to be kind of skillful when you say no—not be too quick to say yes. I think you have to take into account if somebody wants to do something, what effect it's going to have on somebody else, some other service, some other program. You have to take into account what effect it's going to have on [the health science center]. We've tried over the years to dovetail things so that we're not unnecessarily duplicating services. I think keeping an open door and open communication with the medical staff is key.

The Importance of Timely Communication and Follow-Through

From an executive at Leonard Morse Hospital:

> I think accessibility is key. If a doctor wants to see us, it's pretty clear they can. My secretary says that whatever it is, I will make time that day. I've set up meetings with the chiefs on a one-to-one basis and bring them up-to-date on everything going on. I do the same with the board every month in terms of financial status, statistics, what's happening around us.

From a physician at Tucson Medical Center:

> The management team here is very easy to work with. You call them and if they are not in, they will call you back in two hours.

Figure 6.1 Elements of Effective Communication: A Guiding Framework

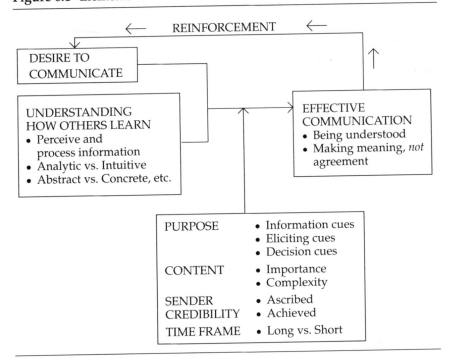

[The CEO] made that mandatory. You will answer any call, even if it's with a "I don't know" answer. When they do that, I know they're being realistic with me. Maybe you don't like what you hear, but they're being honest. They don't act real fast. They may tell you, we're looking into it. If you try to do something first-class, sometimes you don't want to jump feet-first into the river. But when they do something, it's usually been deliberated upon by umpteen committees and board members and they both do first-class jobs. They don't cut corners.

Using Multiple Forms of Communication: Lean and Rich

From a physician at Sutter:

Well, we use general medical staff meetings as rumor control. Any member of the staff can ask any question during open forums. Then, we also have publications in which we communicate with people. We also use a lot of one-on-one.

At McAuley, a medical staff newsletter is used to reinforce communication that has occurred in the medical executive committee and committee meetings throughout the hospital. For example, as part of communicating the importance of a new program involving total quality improvement, the president of the medical staff wrote the following in the medical staff newsletter:

> In order to facilitate maximum medical staff participation in this meeting during the morning hours, the operating room and the emergency room will be closed except for emergencies. . . . In addition, departments will be encouraged to cancel one or more of their monthly meetings so that the total meeting time commitment for physicians for the month will not be unreasonably increased. . . . The medical staff leadership is making a strong commitment to be totally involved in this project. They feel that this particular session will provide an exciting initiation to the project for the entire medical staff. I encourage everyone's participation.

The Importance of Frequent Communication

A physician at West Allis Memorial noted:

> It used to be that we had physicians calling board members directly at their home and telling them what was wrong. I can't remember the last time that happened. People are now in [the CEO's] office telling him about this and that. And he weighs the votes. If he hears something from a lot of people, well maybe that means something. Of course, there's always somebody that doesn't like something, and that has to be discounted. The leadership of the staff communicates very easily with him and vice versa. If the medical staff is aware of a problem, they don't hesitate to share it with administration. The board knows that and is willing to watch and wait. We have a long history of trust. [The CEO] won't lie to the board. And the physicians know [the CEO] won't blindside them.

In a similar vein, a board member at Lexington Medical Center commented:

> We have a history of very close communication among the board, administration, and medical staff. There's never been antagonism. We emphasize straight answers. The chiefs of staff have almost always maintained good communication with the board. They asked us whether we're hearing enough and whether we have any

questions. . . . A lot of really effective communication goes on at retreats. The board joins the medical executive committee on their three-day retreat each year.

A physician at Lexington Medical Center commented:

Administration doesn't bring up things that are entirely new. They are open and up-front all along. It's a breath of fresh air. As a result, we have a "work well together" feeling.

How Communication Builds Trust

From a physician at Tucson Medical Center:

I think it is extremely important that there should be management by walking around. I set this up a number of years ago. We walk around and see if there are any problems. We ask how we can help. In the process, we have avoided a lot of problems. Also, we get to know the nurses and the clerks out there, and they get to know us. They know who they can contact. They appreciate that tremendously. I've gotten good feedback, and they really appreciate that. It hardly takes any time at all and it saves a lot of aggravation. . . . We get back to people with answers to their problems.
    . . . Another thing I would like to see administration do with the staff is to follow through. They listen, but it may be months before they'll follow through. It may be months before they decide to do anything. By that time, clinicians have said they don't care. . . . When they do respond, it seems that it's taken such a long time. Feedback is very important even if you're not going to do something for four or five months. What I do when something's going to happen that's going to be delayed is that I always call people in and let them know. I say I'm still thinking about it, I haven't forgotten you. . . . Personal contact is key to building up trust.

The following passage (Helt 1985) summarizes many of these points. Most importantly, it suggests that communication is an act of commitment to the other person and to the organization.

As individuals working in organizations, we have two basic tools always available to us: our word or commitment to do what we agreed to do, and our ability and willingness to communicate openly and honestly with others. When we give our word, we sometimes take it casually. We give our word to try to do what we promised, and we mean that we will to the extent that all events leading to the keeping of our promise go according to plan. We keep our word to the degree that it is convenient or to the extent that our colleagues provide the right circumstances.

What happens when circumstances make it difficult to keep our commitment? Usually, we produce excuses—we justify our failures to produce the promised result. Again, the cost to our integrity and the effectiveness of the organization is substantial. Once a condition is established where a person's commitment is treated lightly, enormous uncertainty exists in all interactivity. Unwritten rules were introduced, such as it's ok to be late for meetings or work, to leave work unfinished or even unstarted by the promised time. It doesn't take long to create cynicism and disbelief. Furthermore, a situation like this is somehow communicated to clients, customers, competitors, suppliers—all organizations with which we do business. We're now on a downward spiral of no integrity and no results.

The first step to correcting the situation is regaining integrity. This requires vigilance and an uncompromising willingness to be truthful. This is so important that we spend a disproportionate amount of time at Laventhol and Horwath's Managing for Results Program training people to be completely honest in their communication, no matter how uncomfortable it may be. They are trained to promise only what they are sure they can deliver and to list any and all contingencies relating to the commitment. This has tremendous influence on the listener. He is made to believe in the strength of the promise and is alerted to behave similarly when it's his turn to make a promise.

Our training includes focusing on completing communications. Too often managers and other employees withhold communications. They don't say what they want for fear of making someone sad, or mad or because it might seem petty. There are proper ways to deliver sensitive communications, but they should be communicated. Until an environment exists where it is acceptable to speak openly and honestly, an institution will be at an impasse, trying to produce results over a bundle of unmentioned obstacles. While this process of completing formally withheld communications can be very uncomfortable, it can also create a work environment that is enlivening, filled with energy and openness. It can erase hard workers' resentment against goof offs and promise makers who don't deliver, as the openness either inspires people or leads to job termination. Openness is a process that feeds on itself as it lightens burdens.

COMMUNICATION BEST PRACTICES

Listed below are several examples of outstanding communication best practices that may be used to improve hospital-physician communication.

1. The CEO visits medical departments and service chiefs routinely to discuss strategic and operational issues, field questions, and control rumors. The CEO asks for help in managing challenges and does not pretend to always know what to do.

2. The CEO and other members of administration make patient rounds. This helps to maintain visibility and accessibility.

3. Personal one-on-one communication is emphasized. Administrators meet with physicians for breakfast, lunch, or dinner. Specific approaches are tailored to each physician's concerns and interests.

4. Communication protocols are used in working with physicians. For example, specific guidelines are established for

    a. returning phone calls promptly—for example, within two hours

    b. the number of days to solve a problem

    c. how to close the loop on difficult issues and provide feedback to physicians

    d. resolving nursing issues that arise

    Further, when a lot of changes occur, five administrators each call three doctors immediately. Influential doctors that are most affected by the change are targeted. Special breakfast meetings may also be held.

5. Service facilitator groups are established for each important service. These groups consist of approximately 15 to 25 people, including physicians, nurses, and ancillary professionals concerned with each service. They examine issues related to productivity, service integration, emerging technologies, quality, monitoring of competition, and related issues.

6. A system of dyad doctors is used to improve doctor-nurse communication. Dyad doctors are high-admitting physicians who work well with nurses. They are used as a sounding board for new ideas and for working with physicians who have created problems with the nursing staff.

7. Board members, top management, and physician leaders meet with each other in advance of bad news. For example, in cases

where the board may overturn the medical executive committee's recommendation regarding a specific physician's renewal
of privileges.

8. Physician leaders and hospital executives participate in communications training workshops to improve their skills.

REFERENCES

Athos, A., and J. Gabarro. 1978. *Interpersonal Behavior*. Englewood Cliffs, NJ:
    Prentice-Hall.
Daft, R. L., and R. H. Lengel. 1986. "Organizational Information Requirements,
    Media Richness, and Structural Designs," *Management Science* 32:554–71.
Georgopoulos, B. S., T. A. D'Aunno, and R. Saavedra. 1987. "Hospital-Physi-
    cian Relations under Hospital Prepayment," *Medical Care* 25(8):781–95.
Helt, E. 1985. *Managing for Results*. Philadelphia, PA: Laventhol and Horwath.
Longest, B. B., Jr., and J. M. Klingensmith. 1988. "Coordination and Commu-
    nication," in S. M. Shortell and A. D. Kaluzny (Eds.), *Health Care Management:
    A Text in Organization Theory and Behavior*, 2nd ed. New York: John Wiley and
    Sons, 217–64.
Neuhauser, P. C. 1988. *Tribal Warfare in Organizations*. Cambridge, MA: Ballinger
    Publishing.

CHAPTER 7

Building Trust

The demands of the changing health care environment place great strains on the development and maintenance of trusting relationships between hospitals and physicians, as reflected in the comments of a McAuley physician:

> Given today's environment and some of the things that have occurred with the HMO, wanting to have the level of trust that you had five years ago may be setting yourself up for failure. It may not be obtainable in today's environment. Things are not the same here. The ground rules are not the same. The playing field is not the same so that those expectations and perhaps all other things aren't the same.
>
> When I think of trust, I think it means that most of the time someone is going to do what I expect them to do. I can depend on their following through and arriving at conclusions. . . . I can't expect them to do what I want them to do, or I can't expect them to please me or to respond to my needs in the same way that they have in the past. . . . The problems now become more difficult to solve.

These pressures often result in frustration, anger, and fear; and overreliance on structure to solve problems; a lack of acceptance of one's responsibilities; and an inability to facilitate relationships (Gill and Meighan 1988), and yet, almost to a person, everyone interviewed agreed that it was trust that made everything possible.

FORMS OF TRUST

In order to better understand the role that trust plays in the development of effective relationships, it is useful to think about the different forms of trust that exist.

Normative versus Instrumental

Normative trust is based on shared values between the parties involved. Instrumental-based trust is centered on utilitarian exchange principles, "I will trust you if you reward me with things I want" and vice versa.

Creating overarching goals that both parties can commit to is an example of normative-based trust. Institutions with a long-lasting commitment to high quality and service, such as McAuley, Providence, and Crouse-Irving Memorial, could draw on their history and experience in normative ways to build and maintain trust. Respondents said in effect, "Although we have made our share of mistakes, because we think we share the same values and goals, we can forgive each other and pick up the pieces." Some additional examples of normative-based trust are reflected in the following comments of a physician from Leonard Morse:

> Although you don't always agree with many of the administration's decisions, you trust them . . . because you know the decision is in the best interest of the community we're serving.

A Sutter executive noted:

> Physicians honestly believe that management supports quality. The physicians believe that management is quality oriented. That goes a long way toward building trust. Management is open and lives up to its commitments. Management shows that it is not only willing to accept criticism but will change its approach in response to that criticism. Management works hard at bringing the board and the medical staff together.

Some examples of instrumental-based trust are reflected in the following comments. A West Allis physician noted:

> [The CEO] is not intimidated by them [the physicians]. He feels no need to beat them down and feels no need to outsmart them. He is acutely aware that the prosperity of this hospital is tied to the goodwill of the physicians. He knows that antagonizing the physicians is not in his best interest. While that's on a more Machiavellian level, he also generally likes physicians. And he knows we're in it together. He's willing to tell people things. When I became chief of staff, he met with me to say a few things. He lays down some ground rules and one of the things he asks of the new chief of staff is to do what you have to do, and I'll do what I have to do but don't blindside me. And it goes both ways. He doesn't blindside the board or the medical staff.

A McAuley physician noted:

> I think the proof of the pudding is in the tasting. So for the surgeon, it is, are we going to get this piece of equipment? We understand you're behind it. You see the benefit of it and we hope to see it. It's taking the uncertainty out of trying to remove as much of the uncertainty and misunderstanding as possible. . . . I think from the physician's point of view, it is administrative responsiveness. And from the administrative viewpoint, it is that the physicians understand their relationship with each other and there's a level or willingness to be supportive of the hospital.

A North Monroe physician noted:

> I think that trust is based on respecting the goals of the other person. In other words, the private practitioner doesn't want the hospital going outside and bringing in competition, and so the hospital understands and respects the goals of the physician. It's like a marriage, you don't have to have the same goals, but you have to respect those of the other person. And so if in their day-to-day practice they demonstrate a sensitivity and respect for the goals of the physicians on the staff in providing the best care to their patients and understand the economic aspects of their moves, then that's going to build trust. As far as the hospital having trust in their doctors, I guess it's probably the same way as long as the physicians use their hospital fairly and don't send all the losers to one hospital and the winners to another. As long as they're fair, there's going to be trust in the physician's competency. If you've got an incompetent boob in the administration or incompetent physicians, that's going to break down the trust.

The instrumentality of the relationship in business terms is perhaps expressed most candidly by a Scripps physician:

> I think trust has to do with understanding the specific needs of an institution versus the needs of the individual physician, and it also has to do with the understanding of what business decisions are and why they develop in a given way. We would go to [head of the physician organization] and say, "God damn that hospital, they're screwing us again." He'd laugh. It's not screwing you. They're making good business decisions. Why don't you understand that? It's that kind of thought process which is critical. Physicians are not used to thinking in terms of what are good business decisions.
> . . . The trust issue is really understanding. It's understanding the factors that lead a business—and a hospital is a business—

to reach the conclusions that it does to take the positions that it does. If you understand that, then you can begin to rely on the decisions because they fit into a reasonable business-making process. Once you learn that, then the trust comes much more easily because it's not a matter of these guys trying to stab me in the back because they're not. They're simply following appropriate reasonable business decision-making processes. And physicians don't understand that and they think there's something unethical or something unfair, or they get into a personal vendetta. They say, I can't trust those bastards; they said they were going to do this, that, or the other thing and they haven't. Then they go back in and say, what did they really say, what do they really mean, and what are the processes and forces that are affecting them? I think that's probably been the single most important thing.

Most of the study sites used a mix of normative- and instrumental-based approaches to trust. Appeals to the institutions' overarching values and goals only went so far. Understanding the pragmatic economic and professional needs of each party and acting to meet these needs were an essential part of each institution's strategy. Most CEOs recognized that the interdependence of hospitals and physicians was driven increasingly by instrumental-based economic reality as it was by normative-based shared values. Appeals to the head were important, appeals to the heart inspired, but appeals to the pocketbook were often necessary.

Trait-Based, Process-Based, and Institutionally Based Trust

The basis for trust can come from people's traits, processes of interaction, or the authority and formal position that has been institutionalized over time (or, of course, from various combinations) *Trait-based trust* centers on the personal social characteristics of the parties involved. Reliance may be placed on features such as ethnicity, sex, physical appearance, or profession. Comments such as "she looks like she can be trusted" reflect trait-based trust. Similarly, one might ascribe a greater degree of trust to a minister than a used car salesman. *Process-based trust* is focused on two parties' personal experience of successful interaction with each other. As a result of past interaction, uncertainty in behavior is reduced and some degree of predictability established. In *institutionally based trust*, authority and formalization (rules, laws, etc.) substitute for trait- and process-based trust. This generally occurs in exchanges that cover wide geographical and social areas. Institutionally

Figure 7.1   Stages of Trust Development

$$\longrightarrow$$

Trait-Based Trust $\longleftrightarrow$ Process-Based Trust $\longrightarrow$ Institutionally Based Trust

based trust may become particularly important for hospitals and physicians who are a part of national and regional health care systems. However, it is unlikely that institutionally based trust will come about unless a considerable amount of process-based trust has occurred first, which, in turn, may need to be initiated by each party recognizing certain traits in the other that make such interaction seem worthwhile. This suggested sequential flow is shown in Figure 7.1.

Among the study sites, the four most frequently mentioned factors associated with trust were

1. open, honest communication and a commitment to discuss all issues
2. the perception of being fair in dealing with each other
3. execution and follow-through (doing what you say you were going to do)
4. credibility developed over the years

The first two factors—open, honest communication and the perception of being seen as fair—are traits, although based on the experience of past interaction. Execution and follow-through are clearly aspects of process-based trust. Credibility developed over the years can serve as a source of institutionally based trust. Examples of each of these are highlighted below.

Communication. In regard to communication (see also Chapter 6), the following comments of a McAuley physician are pertinent:

> Trust is based on open communication and a willingness to discuss all issues. . . . There also has to be a willingness and ability to put the negative issues on the table and discuss these as well. Education is needed on the different points of view.

A Tucson physician noted:

> Trust is based on open and honest communication. Our physicians will tolerate them telling us something we don't want to hear if we

say it openly and without rancor. I think the willingness of the hospital to listen and to act upon what they hear allows physicians to have a real impact on major decisions. I think our ability to admit when we've been wrong also helps.

A Providence physician noted:

Trust is the ability to talk with each other. And then feel that when something is done, it is done with your full knowledge of it. Even though you might not have agreed with it, at least you knew you had some input.

As previously noted, external pressures place particular demands on trust. At one institution, the CEO was in the midst of a rather major administrative cutback. His comments below are noteworthy:

We went through this reduction yesterday, and I am going to meet with the management staff this afternoon. What I desperately want to say is that it is now behind us. We have done it and it is behind us. But I know that I can't say that because I don't know what the future holds. So I think one of the real important factors here is that we have been dealing with the medical staff to avoid that temptation of making commitments that you can't meet. You know it has to do with accuracy. You have to have some optimism, but you also need to be realistic.

Fairness. A Crouse-Irving Memorial physician noted:

I think [the CEO] is very fair. . . . You will get a fair discussion and fair consideration. . . . He has been very, very fair in trying to hear what physicians were saying whenever possible and trying to see if it could be implemented.

A North Monroe executive noted:

I think trust is built on one's own integrity. If you compromise your integrity with physicians, they are a very unforgiving group. I think you've got to maintain that integrity. You need to try and treat them all as equals. But again, I think you need to live up to what you say you're going to do and be honest. I mean if you're going to screw them, say so. And if it's a no answer and they don't want to hear it, figure out a way to tell them no in such terms that they walk away still feeling not maybe happy about it, but comfortable with that decision. It's how you communicate with your physicians.

A Tucson executive noted:

> I guess it's no different than any other relationship. Honesty, consistency, trying not to create double standards. The double standard issue is probably the tougher one that we haven't sorted out yet because over the years we've tried to treat all members of our medical staff equally. We've never really been totally successful. Some people were probably unhappy because they felt we were giving preferential treatment to someone else rather than themselves. And now that we've created this relationship with the managed care system and with this PHO [Physician Hospital Organization], we're beginning to send signals to other physicians that we're treating others on a preferential basis. Yet we haven't articulated that as a clear statement down to the grass roots of the organization.

Other "traits" that help to promote trust included the development of physician managers who remained clinically active and the use of middle- and upper-level managers with clinical backgrounds and experiences in working with physicians. In the words of one: "Our physician managers have all maintained a significant clinical presence. . . . They know that in the middle of the night I'm helping to take care of some of their patients when I don't have my administrative hat on."

In regard to middle management background characteristics, a McAuley executive commented:

> We don't have any MBA types that are strictly MBA types. We may have practitioners, a nurse or a pharmacist or a social worker who got an MBA, MHA, or PhD, but they were all practitioners before they did this. There's just an understanding and empathy as to what it takes to provide a service. I think it's very, very important, and I think that it separates us from other administrative staffs.

Process-Based. The following statements reflect some of the dynamics involved in process-based trust. In regard to the importance of getting to know each other, a Providence executive commented:

> I guess the first thing that comes to my mind would be experience. In other words, I trust you today because I have known that in the past you have done what you said you were going to do, and we have dealt with each other in a forthright manner in terms of describing what the situation actually is.

In a similar vein, a Tucson physician notes:

> I think trust can only be developed through education and that's
> why it takes time. I think it means educating physicians into the
> . . . total picture of the hospital and its problems and vice versa.
> The hospital has to learn what the problems are and that the doc-
> tor's not just some guy who brings patients in. But what really are
> his problems? And I think that's the basis to me of what I think is
> developing, and I think that's the only way it can be developed.
> . . . I have to know you before I can trust you and that takes time.
> It takes time to see how you react under certain stresses and under
> certain problems. I think that's the basis of the trust which has
> been good [here].

The following statements shed some light on the importance of
follow-through. A Lexington Medical Center executive noted:

> The key for us is backing up what you say. Getting them [the
> physicians] to believe that what we tell them is reliable. They will
> need to see this.

A Sutter physician noted:

> I guess it's results. That if we talk about something and the medical
> staff takes a side and the administration says yes, we can agree to
> do that, then we've got to perform as we agreed. I think that builds
> trust. Whether it's a TV in the doctors' lounge or free lunch on
> Thursdays, a conference on Friday noons, completing the pa-
> thology lab, buying a piece of equipment, or expanding a service,
> we've come to an understanding that this is what we're going to
> do. And if that understanding is met, then I think it builds trust.
> Then you know you can depend on a person.

Another physician commented:

> To me, it's two things. First, I think being available to hear con-
> cerns and gripes. Second and probably the most important is doing
> what you say you are going to do. If you say you are going to be
> involved in decision making, then you've got to mean that and get
> them [the physicians] involved in decision making. I can remember
> when we had a psychiatry department that had a program they
> were going to develop. Somehow, decisions got made without
> psychiatric input. It took me and the [CEO] and others at least two
> or three years to work through all of the paranoia. The rela-
> tionships are now very good. It really took a lot of conscious effort
> to get that back on track.

A North Monroe physician notes:

> I just like them to know what it is they're saying and when they finally make a decision, what they're going to do. I don't necessarily expect them to agree with me all the time. I like to be informed, and I like to see them go through with whatever it is. Whereas I think a lot of doctors and just people in general are probably satisfied when they get their way, and they're unsatisfied when they don't get their way.

In addition to their willingness to follow through, it is also important to indicate why one may not be able to do so. The following comments of a Crouse-Irving Memorial executive reflect this point:

> I think you have to be open, fair, honest and demonstrate the reason you cannot do what you want to do. You've got to lay it out for them. For example, we do not carry malpractice insurance here, and I tell them we cannot do this. I've had to say no probably a dozen times. It's easy to say no because as long as they know you have a good reason for it, they believe you. It's when you don't have a good reason for it that you get into trouble. They know when you start to kid them.

An example of what can happen when follow-through is not perceived to exist and communication is suspect is illustrated by the following physician's comments:

> My own analysis is that I'm not sure that I believe everything he [an administrative person] says. I think he tells me what I want to hear, but I'm not sure that he would tell another party the same thing. . . . I guess my anxiety is that I sometimes lack that element of trust, that what he is saying is really what he is going to do.

Institutionally Based. Examples of institutionally based trust primarily centered on the stability of the top management team. As a result of such stability, physicians came to trust management authority and judgment. As expressed by one individual at McAuley:

> I think a key factor has been stability in the management team. I've been here in this position for 12 years, so people remember what I said. Our chief operating officer has been here 7 or 8 years. The V.P. for patient care services has been here for 9 years. Many of the administrators have been here for 6, 7, 8 years. One has been here for 25 years. So the management team tends to come here and stay. What's positive about that is you don't have a new team coming in

saying, "Well look, I didn't commit to that. This is a new day and I'm going to do it this way." We don't have turnover. Those relationships get built over a number of years.

TRUST AS A TWO-WAY STREET

While most of the examples have treated trust from the perspective of what the hospital did to earn physician trust, both hospital and physician respondents mentioned things physicians needed to do to be viewed as trustworthy by administration. Not surprisingly, they are some of the same things physicians want from hospital executives—honesty, understanding, and follow-through. The following comments are illustrative. A Leonard Morse executive mentioned:

> What we look for from them [physicians] are probably the same things they look for from us. I think we want to be able to feel that they're being honest in what they're saying to us, that they've taken the time to understand what the issues are, that they're understanding it from an organizational perspective rather than just their own individual needs. I think this is a big leap that we need to accomplish at the moment. . . . Community hospitals certainly have the problem of the individual practitioner always putting their own goals out first and having a difficult time merging them with the organization's goals. And when I look at the hospitals, I don't look at it as just the hospital, it is the hospital and staff working together. And some of them are beginning to understand that better.

A Providence physician noted:

> Physicians need to understand and accept the enormous problems that are faced by these people [administration]. And the fact that they have problems that supersede the individual doctors running around people. . . . It's very easy to distinguish between those things that are totally self-serving, such as I want more donuts in the lounge, to those that are truly going to help the hospital, such as I want my patient to get EKG and chest film in relatively close proximity to one another and not a block and a half away. Administrators need to trust physicians that they are not always just looking out for themselves, but in order for this to be the case physicians need to earn that trust.

A Scripps executive noted:

> The physicians I trust are the ones who are predictable in the sense that what they say is what they do. I also don't want them telling

me something they think I want to hear and then go back and do what they know is right. Because we're businessmen, we understand what the economic motives are, and we can relate to the physician that comes in and says, "I'm starting my own CAT scanner in my office because I can make a lot of money." I'd rather him say that to me than not or to say something else and then go do it. So I've grown closer to the physicians that I can trust who tell me when they're going to do something. I can really believe I know where they're coming from and be very candid with them.

THE CHIEF OF STAFF'S AND MEDICAL DIRECTOR'S ROLE IN BUILDING TRUST

The medical director (for those hospitals that had them) and the chief of staff played key roles in building and maintaining trust between physicians and the hospital. In addition to the formal position power that was associated with the responsibilities, they also used their personal qualities of communication and persuasion to build credibility and trust. Almost all acknowledged, however, that the issues were becoming more complex and that it was becoming increasingly difficult to fully disclose information or to even decide what should be communicated to whom and what should not. This is captured well in the following comments from a Scripps physician:

> There is a lot going on lately in terms of the new building and how we plan to compete. And you have to inform enough people so that both sides know what is going on, but there has to be enough trust that people aren't going to say anything to anybody. I have known some stuff for the last four months about some of the building projects around here. I have been trying to facilitate some of the communication between different groups. I have known some stuff that I would dearly loved to have told to a bunch of people who are really getting disgruntled about how things are going and not trusting things. But I couldn't say a thing. Because if I had said something, everyone would have just gone crazy. And one of the problems with being in a medical staff leadership role is sometimes you get perceived as being bought by the administration. You are told things which just can't be made public knowledge, and you have to say to the medical staff that I just can't tell you that but please just trust me. . . . So there has to be a level of trust, there has to be a level of discretion. And that discretion is very important because otherwise the information can't be shared at all.

TRUST IS FRAGILE

All of the study sites experienced ups and downs in their level of trust. In the case of one site, a key physician was initially excluded from an important medical staff executive committee meeting. He was so incensed that it took several months to repair the bond of trust. As expressed by the CEO, "To this day, he still doesn't have the same positive attitude toward management that he did prior to the incident."

In a second case, trust between physicians and the hospital was seriously eroded when the system corporate office to which the hospital belonged took control of an HMO. The physicians thought the HMO was jointly owned by themselves and the hospital. While the physicians believed the hospital acted with good intentions, they felt betrayed by the fact that the hospital could not control or influence the corporate office. As one physician expressed it: "You folks [the hospital] used to be able to control things over there [the corporate office]. Now, we have a sense you can't do that anymore. Are we playing with the monkey or the organ grinder? We feel we've been misused."

These two examples underscore the point that trust must be earned and reearned every day. Every encounter, situation, or problem is an opportunity to repair, reinforce, or enhance trust. The time one spends, how one communicates, how one listens, how one attempts to follow through are critical to the success of ongoing relationships. Understanding the heart, the head, and the pocketbook are all important and legitimate.

A MINICASE

Some examples of the different forms of trust discussed in this chapter are illustrated by the experience of one of the study sites with HMO and PPO developments, as described by the vice president for planning:

> When we were putting the HMO together, we really had an interesting set of circumstances. Before we put the PPO together, we had been kind of monitoring the PPO movement and had been getting vibes from our doctors that they were . . . beginning to really feel the impact of HMOs on their own business. Within the management group we were talking about whether we should in some way begin promoting the idea of a PPO. We kept thinking, well, you know the physicians probably aren't really ready for this. We went into a retreat. During the retreat in one of the discussion groups, the physicians basically said: You know one of the problems with [the hospital] is it's not aggressive enough. Why haven't

they helped us deal with the HMOs? They should be forming a PPO, by God. And out of that a strong recommendation came that a PPO should be started. So the physicians drove the process. It went very well, very smoothly, and we got it up and running.

Shortly after that we got involved in discussions with [a competing hospital] and [a doctor from another area]. We were wondering whether we should be looking at creating some kind of a system. We engaged a consultant who did a little study for us in terms of what things we might do together. It came out loud and clear that each of us really needed to go the next step and form an HMO. By that time all of us had experienced the purchase of a local HMO and the fact that they were willing to bid the hospitals off against each other. When the HMOs formed here, they first contracted with all the hospitals on billed charges. As they got more volume they came back and said, Well, we want a contract with everyone, but we deserve a little bit of a discount now. So we gave them a 5 percent discount. Then they realized that they could really get a discount if they could move patients around, and in one day we lost 10 percent of our general medical surgical work load by not contracting with what was the predecessor to Maxicare. Well, the handwriting was on the wall that unless we had control of the patient base through having our own managed care system, we were at the whim of a significant bed surplus and the willingness of plans to move their patients around.

We thought this situation would present no problems for the physicians. We went back to them and said, You know, we think the PPO is a great idea. We think it will be successful. But it's only going to be attractive to a certain number of employers and among those employers, a certain number of employees. If we really want to capture a larger group of patients, we need to go the next step and form an HMO. Why at that first meeting I thought I was going to be killed. I mean I was worried that I wasn't going to get out alive. We started to meet on a weekly basis and within three weeks they were driving the system again. It took about three weeks for us to go through a process where they came to the same conclusion that we had before, and we all said, let's go, let's go, let's get it done.

And then as we developed the HMO, we decided the best thing would be to bring our PPO and our HMO together. And so we opened up discussions with a multispecialty group without first going back to the IPA board and taking them along to understand why we should do it. I went to the IPA board meeting where there were a lot of clenched jaws. I basically got up and said, Guys, you're right. We screwed up. We should have come back here and talked about it before we made that next step, but let me tell you why we think it's a good idea. And we talked it through, and they said, fine, go ahead and talk to them. And we agreed to what the criteria would be if we tried to do the deal. So I think being willing to go back and say, "no, you're right, we're not doing the right thing here," is important to developing that trust relationship.

A SUMMARY OF TRUST-BUILDING BEST PRACTICES

1. Consideration is given to both normative issues involving shared values and instrumental issues involving legitimate self-interest.

2. Each party respects the other's right to make a decision based on legitimate business criteria.

3. Trust is developed through open, honest communication; promoting a sense of fairness; following through on one's commitments; and developing consistency through ongoing interaction.

4. Promoting stability of the top management team provides a track record of experience for enhancing trust.

5. The chief of staff, medical director, and other physician leaders are used to help develop and maintain trusting relationships.

6. Because trust is fragile, it must be reearned on a daily basis, using every opportunity presented. This involves being willing to take the risk that one's efforts will be reciprocated.

REFERENCE

Gill, S. L. and S. S. Meighan. 1988. "Five Roadblocks to Effective Partnerships in a Competitive Health Care Environment," *Hospital and Health Services Administration* 33(Winter):505–20.

CHAPTER 8

Managing Conflict

Inherent differences between professionals and organizations provide a natural setting for conflict. To this can be added the specific differences between hospital executives and physicians in socialization and training, as discussed in Chapter 1. In recent years, this bed of coals has frequently been set ablaze by the significant changes occurring in the health care environment. These changes have placed increased strain on hospitals and physicians alike.

For the most part, physicians do not view themselves as part of the hospital organization. As shown in Table 8.1, 72 percent of physicians interviewed (most of whom were leaders) believed that the medical staff primarily viewed themselves as a separate unit rather than as a part of the hospital. In contrast, only 27 percent of hospital executives and lay board members interviewed felt the medical staff was a separate unit. Thus, even in institutions with reputations for strong relationships, there is the recognition that these relationships must contend with the perceived separateness of the staff.

TYPES OF CONFLICT

As in the case of communication and trust, it is necessary to examine the different forms of conflict that exist. Each form suggests potentially different managerial approaches. Among the most commonly recognized forms of conflict are those due to (1) personal differences, (2) departmental or group differences, (3) informational discrepancies, (4) role incompatibility, and (5) environmental stress (Whetten and Cameron 1984). In the case of hospitals and physicians, personal differences and departmental differences may occur among physicians, between physicians and management, or between physicians and nurses. As noted

Table 8.1 Medical Staff Primarily Viewed as a Part of the Hospital
Organization or as a Separate Unit?

	Overall	Physicians	Managers and Lay Board Members
Part	30.8%	19.0%	46.0%
	(37)	(13)	(24)
Separate	52.5%	72.0%	27.0%
	(63)	(49)	(14)
Some of both*	16.7%	8.8%	27.0%
	(20)	(6)	(14)

Note: In no hospital did a majority of respondents view the medical staff as primarily a part of the hospital organization.
*Medical staff leaders view it as part, while rest of staff view it as separate.

earlier, conflict between physicians and nurses and conflict among physicians themselves were especially prevalent in the institutions studied. A rather typical example of conflict among physicians is highlighted below:

> We have a real problem with a nephrologist. We have a dialysis center here on site. The leader had an exclusive contract to provide the service. He has three members in the group, and what he did was he booted out the junior guy. Now, strictly speaking under our contract with him, he has a right to do that. Yet, in the medical staff bylaws, there is a clause that says that people like that are entitled to due process when there's a conflict. The real issue was a quality of care issue. It was clearly a problem of interpersonal relationships with these two physicians. What we did was say to the medical staff that this person has an exclusive contract which allows him to do that. What we want you to do is determine whether that is still the right way to deliver care. Is that organizational form adequate or appropriate? Secondly, we want you to assess whether the person acted appropriately on the basis of the dismissal. Was it appropriate in terms of quality of care concerns? If you conclude that is was appropriate, then great. If you think the person acted inappropriately, then you have to decide if it is sufficient enough to get rid of the person. I don't really care who heads the unit. The purpose is to deliver a high quality of service to patients and to have someone that the medical staff can rely on when they refer patients. So you have to make the judgment. To

me, it's a quality of care issue. We need to do a better job of making sure that person has adequate administrative skills.

An example of a hospital-physician conflict over a trauma program is described below:

> The biggest single problem this year has been our trauma program. It has raised some turf issues, some subspecialty coverage issues and problems of compensation. I've probably spent more time trying to solve trauma issues than any single operating issue in the past year. It has a lot to do with the interface with physicians. It's a joint program between ourselves and the university medical center, so it's a dual site delivery system. . . . Right now I could end up losing all of my neurosurgeons if we don't play it right. It has angered our only two pediatric general surgeons, who didn't like the fact that their residents were being used to help support the trauma program. Some of the specialties feel we're giving preferential use of our resources to the trauma program and that somehow we're not balancing our commitment to the rest of them. So we're always trying to maintain that balance, recognizing that there's a certain urgency of response and resource commitment associated with trauma. It can have devastating consequences. If we don't get enough general surgeons to come to the trauma program and have to close it down, the university medical center will be the sole deliverer. Two years from now as they [the university medical center] grow and become successful, our medical staff will say we have lost the cutting edge. This is a big-ticket item for us.

The following comments describe a conflict situation growing out of a joint venture consideration:

> We've had an issue with one of our radiologists trying to capitalize on some research work. He wants to develop a diagnostic prostate cancer center. We wanted to work together in order to establish a prostate program as a cooperative joint venture. But, it raises a lot of questions. We've got two groups of urologists and they can't get together. It's been a continual difficulty. Finally, at the last medical staff executive meeting, we were able to make a decision, which was one of the first ones I've seen them make. They said, "We're going to proceed with this even though we know that one of those groups of urologists is angry and feels disadvantaged." They tried really hard to get it to come together appropriately but just couldn't make it happen, and so they decided to go forward. They did it by secret ballot. It was a 17 to 5 vote to move forward. That is a significant event.

An example of conflict caused by increased environmental stress is noted below:

> I think the things that have caused the most problems over the last two years are conforming to state health department regulations. They've taken up a tremendous amount of time. What I see happening is that in the large and small community hospital, there will be fewer and fewer physicians who will volunteer to take positions as officers of the staff, committee chairmen, and department chiefs as the jobs become more and more onerous. And then I'm not sure what the hospitals are going to do or what the state can do. This is a state that is heading into serious problems. I don't think the state realizes it yet. But I would say ten years from now they're going to find themselves in a very funny position of not having enough senior physicians around here. It's kind of interesting. We've been looking to find somebody in pediatric surgery, but we cannot get somebody to come to [the state]. It's unbelievable. We have the Medicaid system here that is terrible, and the fees for physicians have not been raised since the program was instituted in 1967. So it's a joke. So fewer and fewer people are taking Medicaid patients. The fee system is so low in pediatric surgery we're the only ones between [one city] and [another city] providing the service. The reimbursements are so low that we can't offer people enough money to come here. The malpractice situation is not very good either. But I think when you start putting all these things together, the environment in [city and state] in most fields, and ours in particular, is very bad. So even our own graduates from the residencies here go elsewhere. And I'm sure a lot of other people are going to tell you that. This is going to be a real problem.

In addition, as indicated in Chapters 6 and 7, lack of effective communication and trust can result in informational deficiencies between the groups involved and a lack of understanding of appropriate roles—both of which can create conflict. Conflicts between physicians and nurses are examined in Chapter 14.

Conflict can also be characterized by whether it is hierarchical (i.e., between people or groups in a vertical relationship to each other) or horizontal (i.e., between people or groups at the same lateral level with each other); temporary or long lasting; and procedural (i.e., disagreement over means) versus outcome oriented (i.e., disagreement over the ends or the results achieved)(Theodosian 1989). In general, the ten sites were more successful when the differences between hospitals and physicians could be structured more along horizontal than vertical lines, perceived as temporary rather than institutionalized as long lasting (as expressed by one respondent: "You don't overcome one hundred years of history in two or three years."), and focused on differences in means rather than ends. Some of the approaches that the ten sites used to manage conflict are examined below.

APPROACHES TO CONFLICT MANAGEMENT

There are five basic approaches to managing conflicts: forcing, accommodating, avoiding, compromising, and collaborating (Filley 1975, 1978). Forcing occurs when one or the other person attempts to satisfy their own needs at the expense of the other. Usually the situation is viewed as a zero-sum game, where one person's benefit is perceived to be at the expense of the other person's loss. Multiple methods may be used to force an issue including a person's own formal authority, appealing to a higher authority, or referring the issue to a committee that is likely to rule in favor of the person forcing the issue. While there may be times when issues need to be forced, frequent use of this approach breeds high emotional cost and stifles initiative and creative problem solving.

The accommodating approach satisfies the other person's needs at the expense of one's own. While this may be appropriate in certain situations, it generally leads to bottled-up animosity on the part of the accommodating party, a lack of respect for the accommodating party, and perhaps, most importantly, a less optimal solution to the problem.

The avoiding approach results in conflict being ignored. Occasionally a situation between two or more people or groups may be so intense that problems should be avoided. Also, some problems do go away. But habitually avoiding problems and conflict means that issues never get resolved, frustration levels rise, and what started out as a manageable problem becomes much more difficult to solve.

The compromise approach involves both parties sacrificing some of their objectives to achieve some gain. While this approach is effective in some situations, it seldom results in the best solution to problems. Also, managers who characteristically split the difference with their colleagues or subordinates give the appearance of trying to keep the peace at almost all costs. In these cases, compromise simply represents a higher level form of avoidance.

Collaborative approaches rely on open problem solving among the parties involved. The goal is to find win-win situations that satisfy each party. The search is for the best solution under the circumstances. This approach tends to be the most effective for dealing with difficult problems that do not involve deep-rooted personality conflicts (Phillips and

Cheston 1979). But, this approach also requires time and a reasonably high level of maturity on the part of the individuals involved.

While individuals tend to have natural preferences for one or more of the above approaches, effective managers tend to use a variety of styles depending on the demands of the situation (Downey, Sheridan, and Slocum 1976; Schriesheim and Von Glinow 1977). Among the most important factors influencing the selection of a conflict management approach are (1) the nature of the issue being addressed, (2) the importance of a supportive relationship between the two parties, (3) the nature of the formal relationship between the two parties, and (4) the time pressures involved (Whetten and Cameron 1984). As shown in Table 8.2, the forcing approach is most feasible when the issue involved is very important, a supportive relationship is not important, a superior-subordinate relationship exists, and time pressures are urgent. While the forcing approach can work in some areas of hospital decision making, it is seldom relevant for working with physicians because the supportive aspects of the relationship are extremely important and the relationship is seldom of a superior-subordinate nature. Even where physicians are employed, as in the case of hospital-based specialists, executives are likely to be much more effective if they work with their salaried physicians as professional peers.

The accommodating approach works best where supportive relationships between superior and subordinate or peers are important and where a relatively unimportant issue needs to be settled in a timely fashion. This requires hospital executives and physicians to be able to distinguish important from unimportant issues and to get on with the task. As expressed by one medical staff executive committee member: "We no longer go to the mat anymore on every problem. We've learned to save our energy for what's really important."

A compromise approach is most frequently called for when there are important issues that exist among peers who are in a long-term supportive relationship with each other and where time exists to negotiate the compromise. This approach may be particularly helpful in managing conflict among physicians. Often, physicians' inclinations in such situations are to use a win-lose forcing approach, which only creates more problems.

The collaborative problem-solving approach tends to be the best choice to address important issues involving peers when an ongoing relationship exists and when there is sufficient time to define the problem and explore relevant options. This was the approach most frequently used by hospitals and physicians in the study sites. In fact, in several cases this approach was used even when time pressures were urgent. As a result, opportunities were sometimes lost to faster moving

Table 8.2 Matching Situational Factors with Conflict Management Approaches

| Approaches | Nature of Issue | | Supportive Relationship Needed | | Formal Relationship | | Time Pressures | |
	Important Complex	Not Important Simple	Yes	No	Superior-Subordinate	Peer	High	Low
Forcing	P			P	P		P	
Accommodating		S	P		P	S	S	
Compromising	P		S			S		P
Collaborating	P		P			P		P
Avoiding		P	P				S	

Note: P = primary condition; S = secondary condition.
Source: Adapted from *Developing Management Skills* by David A. Whetten and Kim S. Cameron. Copyright © 1984 by Scott, Foresman, and Company. Reprinted by permission of HarperCollins Publishers.

competitors, but the hospitals were willing to pay the price in order to create a higher level of trust with their physicians (see Chapter 7). The hospitals did not feel they could afford to force such issues.

Finally, avoiding conflict is a reasonable path to explore when dealing with minor problems involving people who need to maintain a supportive relationship with each other and it is important not to lose time over the issue. As one medical staff president commented: "We have some people [physicians] that fight all the time over the darnedest things. I think they actually enjoy it. We mostly just ignore them."

SOME EXAMPLES FROM THE FRONT LINE

Respondents from the study sites indicated that the most frequent approaches used to deal with conflict were

1. working through existing committees and parallel organizations
2. using specifically tailored ad hoc task forces and committees
3. using a lot of one-on-one communication and wide sharing of information
4. resolving issues as low as possible in the organizational hierarchy

Most of these mechanisms were used as forums for collaborative problem solving in the search for common interests and overlapping objectives (Gill 1987).

Collaborative Problem-Solving Approaches

Specific Examples.   An executive at McAuley described the CEO's style in dealing with conflict caused by misinformation as follows:

We try to hit the misinformation head on. [The CEO] has met directly with the surgical coordinating committee on all kinds of things, such as how much money the corporation was taking out of here. Also, they were wondering why it was that administration had a plan under the desk to end up with a czar of surgery. So [the CEO] took those questions, prepared himself well, went to the surgical coordinating committee, and just sat with them and shared information. He passed out financial statements; he passed out the history of how much money was sent to the corporation and all of those things; he explained how we loaned money to some people under various conditions and how it was paid back. It was all very specific information. He [the CEO] is going to each of the departments. . . . Where we stub our toe, I think, is when we don't listen and when we think we know enough and haven't included a sufficient number or the right people from the medical staff in the process. I think that tends to be where we run into problems.

A conflict over determining privileges for physicians at immediate care centers was addressed by Sutter:

We dealt with the issue at our strategy retreat. We had to create a new category of medical staff because the physicians who staff these immediate care centers don't have admitting privileges. This led the medical staff leadership to say, "Hey, why should we be responsible for proctoring their quality assurance when we're never going to see these guys." . . . So we said, "Well, you know we'll just create a department of ambulatory medicine and maybe they can have a seat at the medical executive committee." And the physicians really got upset because they said that the standards would be different from what they are for admitting physicians. They don't have to be board certified, for example. And the doctors said that that's two standards of care and they don't want to be associated with it even though it is Sutter Ambulatory Care Corporation. We finally worked it out. In fact, they're going to be a subset of the Department of Family Practice. But we were almost at loggerheads until one of the trustees, who's a retired Air Force general, made a beautiful observation. He said, "You know, we're all talking about different standards of care. he said, "In the Air Force, there are different kinds of pilots. We've got fighter pilots, and we've got tanker pilots, and we've got cargo pilots." And he said, "They're just different people. You don't say that a fighter pilot is better than a cargo pilot. They're just different." . . . And the medical staff guy said, "You're right, you know." So it changed from a thing of where they looked down their collective noses at these guys out in the immediate care centers and began saying they're just different, and it's o.k. for different standards to apply.

At North Monroe, a sticky problem arose regarding privileges for an ear, nose, and throat (ENT) specialist. The situation was described as follows:

ENT training today is so different than it was ten years ago. We had a bright young ENT person complete his residency, and when he applied for privileges he wanted to do thyroidectomies. Well, the committee said: "Absolutely not! It's never been done before by an ENT person; that's a general surgeon's job. ENT just does ear, nose, and throat." But our credentials committee, even though it's geared more towards the older physicians in composition, decided to look into it further. So I talked to him and asked how many cases he'd done during his residency. He came back fully prepared with a recommendation from the chief of surgery at LSU, and he'd probably done about 140 thyroidectomies. In fact, he'd probably done more than most general surgeons. The credentials committee, after reviewing this documentation, said they would endorse it. It went to the executive committee and they endorsed it and the board endorsed it.

The philosophy of collaborative problem solving at Lexington Medical Center was expressed by one executive:

I [the CEO] meet with the chief of staff a couple of times a week. We don't want any surprises. I also meet fairly regularly with the past chiefs, and we use a lot of committees.

Role Played by Task Forces, Committees, and Parallel Organizations. Several observers have noted the important role that both standing and ad hoc committees or groups, and parallel organizations, can play in managing hospital-physician conflict (Derzon 1988; Bettner and Collins 1987). Several examples from the study sites underscore this point. For example, at West Allis the joint conference committee, made up of board members, clinical department heads, the chief of staff, and the CEO, meets monthly to address the most important conflict issues. As expressed by the CEO: "We try to get things out into the open arenas and forums."

At Sutter, a potentially explosive problem with the orthopedic department was handled in the following fashion:

We averted a disaster when our orthopedic department threatened to not cover the emergency room. We set up a task force that was able to resolve this issue. The task force was able to come up with several ideas on how the department could be covered. The main idea was to form a group that could take the cases, regardless of insurance and who the primary care doctor was. The idea was that the pool would be reimbursed about 80 percent of charges, and it didn't matter that they had to share all the risks. The pool could become a separate entity. The attorneys said it would work. However, when it was presented to the orthopedists, they rejected it. They liked what they got now compared to this proposal. But we made them aware of the facts and figures, that the numbers they were talking about were not that great, and most of those people had insurance coverage. So, they had the data in front of them. The realization that it was not as bad as they thought and that alternatives were not acceptable wasn't true. So at this point, they said they'll wait until they find something better. So at least we averted a deadline that was set by the department.

The importance of ad hoc committees is emphasized by the following McAuley physician:

I think the ad hoc committee approach works well for us. Getting some key people together in a small group who really have researched the problem. You talk with the people and come to a conclusion and then report back. That's an effective way. I think that gets around a lot of the useless debate that can go on in a larger group.

The importance of handling issues at the right level and with the right types of committees is highlighted by a North Monroe executive:

Of course, it depends on which level you're dealing with. You have to involve people in the decision making at the right level. Typically, we'll have department heads get together to try to figure out the solution to the problem, and then they may go back to their specific departments and determine how that will apply specifically to that one area. If it's a level that we feel is of a confidential nature, then we won't involve the entire staff, but will primarily work with administration and certain key physicians. Typically, we call people in or go to their office and just discuss it and try to figure out what the root cause is. We try to involve people who are most knowledgeable about the problem. And when we talk about the alternatives . . . we try to use the best alternative. We then implement it and monitor it to see how good the decision was. Did it work, was it effective, was it the best alternative, or should we try another alternative?

The role that a parallel organization such as a physician-hospital organization can play is highlighted by a Tucson executive:

We use the PHO as a forum where almost anything is fair game. I mean if we want to put something on the table that we feel may be sensitive to physicians, that's where we put it on the table. We visit over an issue or an idea and get feedback from them. I think they have found that it's not a sterile exercise knowing that we're not going to do any damn thing we want. I think they understand that if they don't think it is a very good idea, the chances are that it's not going to happen. We bring issues to that forum before they become problems. They'll ask questions about things that they have heard and we do it in a nonthreatening way. It's a very significant mechanism.

The positive role that a joint nurse-physician committee can play is emphasized by a Leonard Morse executive:

We've set up a nurse-physician committee which is made up of what we hope to be some physician leadership and a blend of nursing leadership and administrative staff. Our hope is that the committee will begin to not just react to the day-to-day operational issues but to really stop to talk about what is changing. We need to understand the changes necessary in order to go forward. It's very nice to sit there and say you can't change this and you can't change that. We just can't do everything the same way. The quality of care doesn't necessarily have to go down, but we have a lot of things around here that if reallocated would allow us to provide a very significant amount of resources to the nursing area. We've got to manage the change in order to do that.

The importance of making sure that problem-solving committees are well coordinated is emphasized by a Tucson Medical Center physician:

Our committees interface very well with each other. The lines of authority are all looked at on an ongoing basis, and we sometimes change the lines of authority as issues change. For example, we had an emergency committee that was responsible for the department of surgery's schedule. But that really wasn't appropriate because there is so much more going on in the emergency room. So now they have an enlarged emergency committee which includes everything to do with emergency services, and that reports directly to the medical executive committee. Occasionally, these things have occurred historically, and we have to review them to see whether or not they continue to be right.

An executive at Sutter highlights the importance of good advance committee work with the following comments:

We use a lot of ad hoc committees, and we have a very functional committee system both at the board level and medical staff level. The committees really do work hard so that by the time that things come either to the medical executive committee or to the board, there is a recommendation. One of the characteristics of our work is mutual respect and collegiality. The two organized bodies share this in common. A recommendation surfaces through the committee structure rather than beating it to death or people nit-picking it that weren't on the committee. The style of both bodies is for the leader chairman or the chief of staff to sense that there's not going to be consensus around the issue. We refer that to a subcommittee to work on it further. You get your problems done there rather than spending the group's time. That's a joy.

And the way in which prior informal discussion can help to diffuse issues is indicated by a North Monroe executive:

Prior to meetings there are important critical issues where there could be some confrontation or adversarial relationships. I try to do a lot of politicking behind the scenes prior to those meetings so that everyone is informed of all positions. And many times you can diffuse a lot of controversy in these meetings by doing your homework and talking to the participants behind the scenes. And I think that's true not only in medical staff relationships and board relationships but problem solving in general.

In reviewing these comments and considering the interview materials at large, an overall pattern of one-on-one communication and use of committees emerged. In general, one-on-one communication was used when there was a relatively simple problem involving a single individual. In these cases, the chief of the medical staff or the section head would usually speak with the individual involved. For conflict that involved more than one person or departmentwide issues, different approaches would be taken. If the problem was reasonably well structured, then it was referred to an existing standing committee. They usually dealt with quality assurance, credentialing, new technology requests, budgeting, and related issues. The mechanisms used also varied by hospital size. Smaller hospitals primarily used one-on-one communication and the standing committee structure. Larger hospitals used these mechanisms but also supplemented them with ad hoc committees, task forces, and parallel organizations. Coordinating the various mechanisms for processing conflict was a particular challenge for the larger institutions. If the problem involved a new issue requiring new data collection and analysis, ad hoc committees were frequently used. Examples included emergency room on-call coverage, coverage for trauma services, referral lists, and exploring new managed care contracting opportunities. Finally, the joint conference committee, or a similar group such as a physician-hospital organization, was used to deal with lingering problems that could not be handled through the existing committee structure or through ad hoc special task forces.

Involving the Right People. A difficult surgery schedule problem was resolved at Scripps by involving the right people. As explained by a Scripps executive:

> We've got a lot of problems right now with our surgery schedule. It's computerized and not going well. So we formed a task force of physician leadership and management, and the discussion's going beautifully. Everyone is excited and they're involved. There is a tremendous amount of ownership that people take in this organization. If something doesn't work, they all take it personally. I would say surgery scheduling is a good example of where if we have a problem, we can identify the problem halfway through the solution. Then if I can get the right people surrounding that problem and talking, it really takes care of itself. It's just a question of how many times they have to meet to really solve it and a question of getting the right people involved. . . . This approach also worked with our trauma problem. I'd say that's where we all learned that if you put the right people together, it has an incredible synergistic value. So far, knock on wood, we're the only hospital that has gone through the trauma issue and kept its administrator. All the others have had turnover for other reasons, but certainly trauma was one of the reasons. It can work really well for you if you know how to work with physicians or, if you don't, it can destroy you. I'm convinced of that.

The importance of getting the right people involved is also addressed by a McAuley executive:

> The successes have been where we have picked the right people in terms of involvement. Where you get people that have influence as leaders. The big mistake is when we've got the wrong people involved. We haven't sorted things out carefully enough or determined who the people are that have the biggest problem. I've seen it happen here where you want to do something so badly, but you only ask the people that already agree with you. . . . Our big success stories are where we have properly identified the people that are going to have the most difficulty with that decision.

At Crouse-Irving Memorial the right people are involved through a series of coordinated committees, as described by the CEO below:

> Probably the main committee is the executive committee of the medical staff. Basically, if I have a problem, I will first sit down with the president of the medical staff and the chief of the service and see what differences we have. If we can't work it out, we'll

then cut across two or three services to see if that works. If we need more help, we'll then go to the medical executive committee. There's sort of an agreement beforehand that if we can't work it out, that's where it will go. If we can't work it out there, then we'll usually call in the joint conference committee. And we also have a liaison committee to deal with problems between us and the Health Science Center.

Some Special Approaches. At McAuley, collaborative conflict management and problem solving is encouraged through a service line manager approach. This approach is described by a hospital board member as follows:

> In surgery, I think our service line manager approach has helped in resolving some of the conflict. One of the things that we've been able to do is get the issues on the table in committees and in work groups. We do a lot of listening, and feeding back what we're hearing. The service line managers are there to work with the physicians to get the services to the patients in the best way possible.

At North Monroe an administrative morning report serves as a useful forum for nipping conflict in the bud. As described by the CEO:

> A lot of ideas are generated in the morning report. I just can't emphasize that enough; that's so helpful to us. We do a lot of brain-storming in there, a lot of soul-searching. For instance, about five or six months ago the competition went up on their shift differentials for nurses, and that's a significant amount of money for us. There is no way that we could compete with that. So we got together with a lot of people's help and came up with an alternative benefit package. . . . I've yet to lose a nurse to another facility.

At Providence, an in-house counsel is used to promote due process and provide relevant information for problem solving. As described by one physician:

> We've had a couple of physicians we've had to deal with. We're all fearful of due process and of getting into problems. . . . We have an in-house counsel, who's office is here. I asked her the other day how many problems we have. Other hospitals have to call to get advice and information how to handle things. But we can just take things straight to [name of person] and we get an informed opin-

ion. The information she provides helps us enormously in our credentialing process and review process.

Role Played by Medical Staff Leadership

A key factor in effective conflict management for the study sites was the role played by medical staff leadership—both by the medical executive committee and the medical director (for those institutions that had medical directors). In this regard, a McAuley physician noted:

> I have been . . . pleased about the ability of the medical staff leadership to look at issues from the viewpoint of the good of the institution rather than their own parochial point of view. That does not need prodding; it simply comes out, and it's really helpful when you're dealing with difficulties. I think that's probably the outcome of participation by the leadership in discussing the issues over the years. They have come to understand the importance of the institutional perspective.

At North Monroe, a board member shared the following example:

> We had a situation in which we had some top surgeons that weren't filling out their reports, so we had to advise them that they couldn't work in the hospital until they got their business back together. That was a little bit of a problem. . . . Our chief of staff [doctor's name] handled it in a very professional manner. He met with the physicians and got it worked out.

A board member at Crouse-Irving Memorial highlights the role played by its medical director in resolving conflict:

> Whenever we have an incident in the hospital, he [the medical director] works with the vice president of nursing to investigate it and report it to the board. He works on many of the disciplinary problems. I call him sort of an "arbitrator" who tries to find ways to resolve problems. He works with the chiefs of the departments and their problems. He's an excellent person to work with the administration and the physicians in trying to be a good arbitrator.

A Providence board member indicated the importance of strong medical staff leadership as follows:

> One of the things we do here is to depend on our medical staff leadership. I meet every week for an hour with the past president, the president, president elect, and the other board members to talk about issues that are going on. Out of that comes decisions and directions as well as the exchange of information. . . . For example,

right now we are dealing with planning a medical staff and administration day and a half retreat to provide an overview on some issues. We are also using medical directors more. We have a strong medical director for the hospital, and we also have strong medical directors for certain services. We have medical directors at all the clinics, and we are trying to pick strong people who are involved in managed care and have part ownership in a managed care effort. And so, medical staff leadership is brought into that.

An example of medical staff leadership at Tucson Medical Center indicates the handling of one-on-one situations:

> Most of our issues are resolved simply on a physician-to-physician basis. You can get almost anything done that needs to be done that way. If there's a surgeon, for example, who's doing a particular kind of case that everybody pretty much agrees he shouldn't be doing and he's had a couple of complications, we have the chief of surgery call him up and say, "Hey, you know, is this something you really want to be doing? If you really do, then we're going to have to investigate it and see what your level of complications is." Historically, that's all that's been necessary. The guys say that they don't need that kind of hassle. And I think as a medical staff we've been pretty successful at taking care of problems on that kind of basis.

What Happens When Problems Do Not Get Resolved?

Despite the prevalence of collaborative problem-solving approaches, conflicts were not always resolved. For example, a major problem existed for hospitals that had a split medical staff that could play off one hospital against the other. One example is provided by the comments of a Providence physician:

> I think that a bad aspect of having physicians on two staffs is that the physicians won't spend enough time or energy to command and push through something that is in the interests of this institution. For example, if I say I'd like to see the chart changed, I have to go to the committee and I talk to them and I say it. And the head of the medical records might say we can't do that. And I say, But you need to do it; it's done elsewhere. And he says, I can't do it, then the hour's up and I go and practice somewhere else. The next time I have a problem or conflict, I take my patients somewhere else. I don't have the time or energy to fight this individual, particularly when I know he's wrong because it's being done differently elsewhere, and that's happening here.

When not effectively resolved, issues can also spill over into other areas of the hospital-physician relationship. An example is provided by a Crouse-Irving Memorial physician:

> We had a situation where a physician brought a lawsuit against us. . . . I think it spilled over into a lot of areas of the medical staff because when something like this comes up, you know the entire medical staff gets very paranoid about it. And so a lot of people got very concerned, and they wondered whether they were going to have any problems. Is it going to happen to them? Obviously, it doesn't have to and it hasn't, but it was a real problem for this particular physician and attorney. The chief of anesthesiology is a hospital employee so, therefore, the hospital got branded. . . . I think that caused some of the problem.

Sometimes it is necessary to turn to more formal dispute resolution techniques such as arbitration, mediation, facilitation, and fact finding. These approaches are likely to be most successful when the parties involved have an established ongoing relationship and anticipate continued relationships in the future (American Hospital Association 1988).

PRODUCTIVE VERSUS UNPRODUCTIVE CONFLICT

What Works

Conflict will continue to increase as an everyday fact of life in American health care organizations. Effective executives find ways of actively managing, channeling, and structuring the conflict in productive directions. Based on the experiences of the ten sites and existing literature, there appear to be six important characteristics of productive conflict.

1. *Problem-centered focus.* In the examples discussed, one is struck by the extent to which the primary focus is on solving the problem rather than dealing with differences in personality or extraneous circumstances. The focus is largely on problem-centered complaints rather than person-centered criticism.

2. *Minimization of personality differences.* Effort is made to promote the common ground and the interdependency between the hospital and the physician. Specialty differences among physicians are recognized but are not attributed to personal individual problems or orientations. Physicians are given opportunities to work out the problem themselves, and where this cannot be done, the medical staff and hospital leadership then take appropriate action. Medical directors play a key mediating role.

3. *Full information disclosure.* Efforts are made to bring relevant information to bear on the problem. Physicians respond to facts, data, and analysis. Efforts are made to engage all the relevant parties in the issue, and everyone shares perspectives.

4. *Production of new ideas.* Open collaborative problem-solving approaches provide the opportunity to be creative. There is little pressure to set artificial deadlines or look for immediate solutions to problems that require further investigation. Efforts are made to ensure that the work of different committees is integrated. Committees do not get bogged down in trivia.

5. *Support of ongoing relationships.* The hospitals and physicians involved recognized that they will be living with each other in the long run. Thus, ways were found to deal with problems that minimized negative fallout. Attempts were made to balance various considerations.

6. *Reach for excellence.* The parties involved tend to look for approaches that will challenge the best in each other, to come up with the most creative approaches (see number 4 above) and solutions that will set standards for future problem solving. The most knowledgeable and interested people are involved.

What Does Not Work

Based on the sites' experiences there are also a number of approaches that do not work.

1. *Moving too fast.* Sites frequently got into trouble when they attempted to move too quickly. They were generally better off waiting to make sure the key parties were aboard, even if this meant slower implementation of desired strategies.

2. *Not involving the right people.* It is particularly important to involve physicians who are against the idea. They need to be heard even if their viewpoints are not ultimately adopted.

3. *Not providing sufficient information.* Incomplete or distorted information provides additional ammunition for disruptive conflict. Participants need to believe they have equal access to relevant data and information.

4. *Failing to clarify committee roles.* Physicians need to know where to take various issues. The role of each committee and task force needs to be clarified, as well as the relationships among the committees.

5. *Placing too much responsibility on a few physician leaders.* It is better to reduce the number of significant issues to be addressed than to overburden a few dedicated physician leaders. Managers must shape the set of strategic issues facing the hospital to the capabilities of the staff to deal with them.

6. *Failing to address issues at the appropriate level.* The medical staff executive committee needs to resist being the dumping ground for problems that should be solved at the department or section level. The executive committee must also recognize the importance of task forces and special subcommittees in dealing with complex problems.

7. *Not directly confronting problems.* Stevens notes that during the 1950s the primary characteristic of hospitals was "conflict avoidance and expansionary drift" (1989, 240). Some problems do go away temporarily but often reoccur in a more severe and complex form. The challenges facing hospitals and physicians today cannot be downplayed.

A MINICASE

A concept developed at Tucson Medical Center, called service facilitator groups, serves as a concluding example. It illustrates many of the effective approaches to conflict management discussed in this chapter. The concept is described by an executive in the following quote:

> We have a process which I call service facilitator groups. This is a concept I developed a couple of years ago based on watching the outcome of a VIP [value improvement program] process, which is a productivity program that brought a multidisciplinary focus to bear on how we could provide a particular product at a lower unit cost. Well, the doctors really got involved in that because they saw things happening. I took that model and created what we're now calling service facilitator groups. We have eight or nine of these. The very first one was in cardiac services and then in women's services. We also have one in oncology and in lasers. They average somewhere between 15 and 25 people. I appointed a chairman who is either a staff or management person in the hospital and then we invite disciplines that impact on that particular service. These may include the business office or nursing or the ancillaries or the physicians. They're all invited to be a member of the group and are told that they are a constituency representative. This is not a committee. They are a group. They are to look at the service for which a group has been formed, and they examine several things.

One is the issue of productivity. Are there ways to do things more efficiently? Second, they are asked to look at the range of services and not just have a narrow vision of the hospital. Are we doing enough on the prehospital or posthospital side? Third is the issue of education. Are we providing the right kinds of education and information to our physicians? Patients? Patients' family? The employees and the environment? Fourth, are there technologies that we ought to be aware of that can potentially impact that service? Fifth, we monitor where the competition is so that we can become a center of excellence as it relates to that particular service. They meet regularly and if they decide that they don't ever want to meet again, they can disband. They have the right to do that. They are not to have any minutes. What they're supposed to do is to make the existing structure of the organization work for them so that a doctor knows what medical staff committee to go to for help. And we've got a number of physicians who are involved in these efforts. Some good things have really happened. Our laser service group, for example, in the course of the last two and a half years has generated nine significant ideas. We now have a national symposium for lasers in which we bring in speakers from foreign countries. They're just doing all kinds of phenomenal things. The doctors on that committee are really charged up. That group has pushed us forward, and we're in the process of building a fixed imaging room and are operating a brand new facility to do vascular laser intervention. So these are the kinds of things that begin to emerge from this particular process.

The service facilitator concept, in addition to serving as a forum for managing conflict, also plays an important role in managing change, a topic addressed in the following chapter.

REFERENCES

American Hospital Association. 1988. *The Report of the Task Force on Dispute Resolution in Hospital–Medical Staff Relationships.* Office of Legal and Regulatory Affairs, Legal Memorandum #13, Chicago, IL, August.
Bettner, M., and F. Collins. 1987. "Physicians and Administrators: Inducing Collaboration," *Hospital and Health Service Administration* 32(May):151–60.
Derzon, R. A. 1988. "The Partnership Between Physicians and Hospitals: Options for Improvement," *Frontiers of Health Services Management* 4(Spring):4–19.
Downey, K., J. Sheridan, and J. Slocum. 1976. "The Path-Goal Theory of Leadership: A Longitudinal Analysis," *Organizational Behavior and Human Performance* 16:156–76.
Filley, A. C. 1975. *Interpersonal Conflict Resolution.* Glenview, IL: Scott, Foresman, and Co.

———. 1978. "Some Normative Issues in Conflict Management," *California Management Review* 71:61–66.

Gill, S. C. 1987. "Can Doctors and Administrators Work Together?" *Physician Executive* (September-October):39–44.

Phillips, E., and R. Cheston. 1979. "Conflict Resolution: What Works," *California Management Review* 21:76–83.

Schriesheim, C., and M. Von Glinow. 1977. "The Path-Goal Theory of Leadership: A Theoretical and Empirical Analysis," *Academy of Management Journal* 20:398–405.

Stevens, R. 1989. *In Sickness and in Wealth: American Hospitals in the Twentieth Century*. New York: Basic Books.

Theodosian, T. 1989. Ernst and Young, Chicago, Il. Personal communication.

Whetten, D. A., and K. S. Cameron. 1984. *Developing Management Skills*. Glenview, Il: Scott, Foresman, and Co.

CHAPTER 9

Managing Change

Change is a process of making things happen. As Lewin (1951) suggested many years ago, change occurs when the forces pushing for it are greater than those pushing against it. As noted in the previous chapter, hospitals and physicians frequently find themselves pushing against each other. This weakens their collective ability to resist undesired changes being pushed by the external environment (for example, third party payers, regulators, competitors, etc.). When hospitals and physicians are able to work together, they can become a proactive force for creating constructive change. They are better able to create their desired environment and future. Thus, establishing an effective working relationship has a double advantage for hospitals and physicians: it helps to reduce their vulnerability to the effects of outside forces and it increases their ability to achieve mutually desired objectives.

TYPES OF CHANGE

Change may be planned or unplanned, and within each may be considered as technical, transitional, or transformational (Kaluzny and Hernandez 1988). Planned change involves a predetermined intention to alter a current situation or state of affairs. For example, a hospital may choose to change from recruiting specialists to recruiting primary care physicians. Unplanned change involves unintended, unanticipated, spontaneous alterations in a current situation or state of affairs. A newly recruited director of an ambulatory surgery center may depart from the hospital's strategic plan for the center by choosing to emphasize cosmetic surgery. Often changes in the hospital's external environment will cause unplanned changes.

Whether planned or unplanned, change may be dominated by technical concerns, involving means but not ends. For example, the development of a new ambulatory surgery center by a competitor may cause a hospital to change the way in which it markets its own ambulatory surgery center. Change may be also of a transitional nature, in which the ends change but not the means. For example, the goal of a hospital's primary care satellite clinic network may change from a break-even financial status and generator of hospital referrals to becoming a money-maker in its own right. The means have not changed, but there is now a new goal to be achieved. Change may be also of a transformational nature, involving both means and ends. The development of a joint physician hospital organization to pursue managed care and diversification opportunities is an example of transformational change.

Of the above types of change, transformational change is the most pronounced and, therefore, the most difficult to manage because both means and ends are involved, resulting in a lack of rootedness in current structure, processes, practices, goals, objectives, and even values. For the most part, the evolving relationship between hospitals and physicians involves transformational change, which places tremendous demands on hospitals and physicians alike. The traditional narrowly defined clinical relationship between hospitals and physicians is being redefined to include a variety of business, economic, and ethically driven issues, requiring a much different structuring of the means. Instead of using the traditional medical staff organization to address the issues, alternative parallel structures, such as IPAs and PHOs, are being used. Because so many of the changes affecting the hospital-physician relationship are of a transformational nature, it is particularly important to understand the processes involved.

THE CHANGE PROCESS

The previous chapters examining managerial style and decision-making involvement, communication, trust, and conflict management have shed considerable light on how the study sites manage change. The lessons, examples, and guidelines from these chapters may be organized around five steps for successfully managing change:

1. creating the need for change
2. creating a new desired vision
3. taking the first steps

4. providing ongoing support
5. managing the pace of change

Creating the Need for Change

A problem faced by many sites was that while the hospital recognized the need for change, many of its physicians did not. People do not change unless they are uncomfortable enough with the status quo, or the rewards from changing are so great, tangible, and attainable that everyone sees the merit in changing. Many physicians were simply not hurting enough to try new approaches. The strategy of most hospital executives was to work with a nucleus of physician leaders to move in desired directions. Hospital and physician leaders frequently made appeals to the external environment in trying to communicate the need for change to other physicians. A Providence physician commented:

> We are under such an economic crunch, I kind of believe in the model of creative tension. You don't really do anything good until you have to. And we are getting to a point where we are going to have to. We are either going to have to figure out how to communicate and do a better job, or we'll come apart even further. Either one could occur.

A Sutter physician noted:

> A lot of our changes involve specific joint ventures with the hospital in trying to compete with Kaiser in some way. . . . I think they are going at it in a very sane way and that they are trying to do it as openly as possible. Right now there are so many doctors who don't want to have anything to do with capitated medicine. So, basically, they're throwing it open to everyone and only a few will come forward.

A North Monroe board member commented:

> Times change. If there's anything so sure as what's going to happen, it's going to be one word—change. This is a different point in time, and you have to tell physicians that when you came here apparently you didn't need help. But now we have young men that spend a lot of time and money getting through medical school, and they need help. They need it more than you needed it when you came here. Also, hospital policy changes and the needs of physicians change. These include money needs. This is what we need to tell some physicians who are objecting to what we're currently doing to recruit new physicians.

One of the most difficult things for any organization to do is to change before it absolutely needs to, as reflected in the following comments of a McAuley physician:

> Whining about something never helps. You've got to see a fairly immediate threat before you're going to change very much. I don't want to change. I hate to change. And if I can sneak by for a while, I probably will. But I think the organization will make the move in time to salvage things. I happen to have a fairly grim view of where I see medicine going. The environment has decided to do what I can't do to organize. There's only one customer. Once there's only one customer, I really have no power. I've already admitted that it's happened. There are basically consortia of industries through insurance companies and the government. They're looking at their costs, and they want to get them down. I guess if I was running the country, I'd like to see them do it, too. So they're going to grind the thing down. I think the individual physician like myself has absolutely no chance. I'm not just talking about the economics of it. You might as well admit that you're not going to be an independent professional. I think the current critical issue for the medical staff is the fraying and crumbling of the primary care base. They're undersupported economically . . . and it may be too late already.

In the process of creating discomfort and dissatisfaction with the status quo, it is also important for executives to recognize the sense of loss that many physicians have in regard to new practice styles and the new health care environment (Gill and Meighan 1988). As expressed by Dr. Al Schultz, vice president of medical affairs at Health One in Minneapolis (American Hospital Association 1988):

> Doctors are angry and depressed. . . . The older ones are waiting to get out. . . . All the factors have led to tremendous distrust among physicians of anything that smells of management and control. . . . That is where the physician manager can help. He can begin to establish physician rapport and can begin to establish trust between doctors and hospital managers.

Inability to create the need for change was among the biggest stumbling blocks for some study hospitals. For example, a Leonard Morse executive noted:

> I think there is a lot of resistance to change, and I think a lot of it has been our inability to successfully implement change. We need to sell it and why it needs to be done.

Creating the Desired New Vision

It is not sufficient to be satisfied with the current state of affairs. It is also necessary to have a vision of the desired new state. Many of the study sites struggled in trying to communicate a clear vision of a desired future state. For most this was done through the strategic planning process (discussed in Chapter 5). This largely involved repositioning the hospital and its physicians to deal with the new competitive environment and the increased demands for performance accountability. It frequently involved the use of alternative organizational structures such as a joint physician hospital organization or independent practice association. The challenge was in trying to communicate a common future state. The key was in linking the physicians' economic and professional interests to those of the hospital. The central focus was on maintaining and increasing the number of patients to be served. This economic objective then had to be linked to the professional objective of maintaining and improving the quality of services. The key ingredient was persuading relevant individuals that the way in which to compete and succeed was based on the quality of care provided. Sometimes, symbols were used to communicate the underlying values desired. For example, as described by a Providence physician:

A new auditorium is something that many of us have felt very strongly about for a long period of time. We need to get a group of physicians in here to advertise the hospital and to have gatherings in a presentable auditorium. This would be an enormous boon to the institution. We all want it. We think that it is more than just a simple symbol; it is a very meaningful symbol.

Some of the difficulty in creating a common vision is well expressed by a McAuley executive as follows:

In terms of economics the point of tension is whether the current IPA can evolve into a different organization and whether the numbers are going to hang in there or, alternatively, whether there are going to be some new primary care groups formed who will dominate and the specialists will work for them. Our approach is to get the people in there and have a retreat. . . . For example, we are talking about surveying the medical staff to see if they will sponsor it. We need to identify the problem areas and what the long term issues are, and we will use the retreat to begin to process that. Again, I would like to get the leaders in a room and start to do some envisioning. . . . What do you want it to be like in five or ten years? And then let's put together a strategic plan to get us there. So that's going to be our approach.

The result of this discussion is described in greater depth in the minicase that concludes this chapter.

Taking the First Steps

Change efforts often falter due to ineffective implementation. In the study sites examined, considerable emphasis was given to implementation. Most of the study sites recognized what was required in regard to commitment, resources, new behaviors and attitudes, new roles, and the ability to experiment with different approaches. Some of these are highlighted in the following comments. A McAuley physician noted:

> What people don't realize . . . is that it's wonderful to find all these problems and then to say well here's how you solve them. You just go out there and ask for more money and just tell the hospital we're the doctors, and you just gotta help us out. But there are about sixteen zillion other meetings that go on before you ever get to that point. I mean there are policies and procedures. It is the trench work involved. Folks love to sit at tables and expound on these wonderful problems and these wonderful solutions, but when you get down at the table and start working on it, it is dirty day in and day out routine. Staff work is what gets the job done. It was the Gorbachev/Reagan meeting that made the TV, but they didn't count the two and a half years that everybody spent making it happen. Those are the people that should get the credit, not the people that do the pontificating.

A Tucson physician commented on problems in bringing specialists and primary care physicians together as follows:

> We're in the process of trying to work on attitudes, and it is more than just the medical staff, it's also the nurses. Nurses reflect doctors' attitudes, and we really have not had much support here for the family practitioner. . . . We need to talk to them in ways that make them feel comfortable. And then we need to talk to the specialists and share with them some of the possibilities. We then need to try and bring these two groups together. Whether or not this is going to be successful I don't know, but at least we are identifying these issues and the processes that we need to go through.

The difficulties involved in changing from the old world to the new world of health care delivery are reflected in the following Tucson executive's comments:

> One of the things we have been talking about for the last couple of years is what we call moving from the old world to the new world. We have this plan for the emergence of our own health care delivery system. But in the meantime, how do you relate to all of the other things like managed care plans? So, one of the big problems we have had with the physicians in the last year is when to contract with other managed care systems in the local community, and when to terminate those. There have been some very stressful negotiations. We have one HMO that is responsible for about 10 percent of our business. About 90 percent of their business is coming to our place as a result of contracts that we negotiated about three years ago. Every time they come to the table they push hard for no increases. This year they wanted a 15 percent decrease from the year before at a time when their utilization of resources on a per day basis was actually increasing. So it gets pretty stressful when these folks come and say, "Well, we're going to take our 10,000 or 12,000 days somewhere else." This has a ripple effect on the organization because the medical staff wonders what will happen if we lose those patients. Others also wonder if we are going to have layoffs.

Some practical first steps are enumerated by a Providence physician in the following comments:

> I guess we have to speed up the problem-solving process. We have to get the people who make the decisions together on a regular basis and solve the issues. In terms of the issues with physicians, I think a couple of things would really be good. I think one of them is that the physicians who are here on the medical staff would do well to form some sort of independent organization, not necessarily to deal with hospital-physician issues, but to deal with the hospital insurance company issues as a group. In this way the physicians as a group and the hospital as an organization could deal with individual third-party members so both the physicians and hospital were happy or could accept the settlement. One of our toughest issues is to know who is really committed to the institution among the physicians. We're in a situation where there are two fairly good size clinics that provide the bulk of our specialty care and they have privileges at both hospitals. It is difficult to

know their commitment to the institution. . . . As a result it is a little difficult for the administration to try and plan for the whole medical staff. I don't know how we are going to do that. It is kind of a strange position to be in, but I suspect that is not unique.

The role of experimentation is described by a Leonard Morris executive below in regard to changes in nursing practice:

> We went through a lot of conversation about how nurse managers have to be very different than they were in the past. So we finally had an agreement that we would have a trial on one of our nursing units where we would call it the experimental unit. We acknowledge that everything on that unit is going to be very different and the measure of success will be first of all if the patients think that their care is good. The physicians will recognize that care is better than it was in the past and the nurses will be satisfied with this model practice and our other criteria. So when this happens we know we have something that works well. And they [the physicians] are allowing it to happen. Fortunately, we were able to put the right people in there so that changes are taking place. Everybody seems to think things are going in the right direction. So we are starting very small.

Providing Support

Changes seldom proceed as planned. The health care environment is too turbulent and people's abilities to deal with changes are too variable to expect consistent implementation. As a result, there is need for ongoing support that recognizes the possibility of additional resources and alternative pathways to the goal. The process is essentially one of recognizing "change within change" and incorporating the flexibility to make continuous adjustments. This need for continued attention and support was recognized by most of the study hospitals. They created forums for support through the committee structure, frequent retreats, and involvement in the strategic planning process, as described in previous chapters. In addition, some hospitals set aside special funds for this purpose. For example, as described by a Leonard Morse executive:

> We think that forming a physician-hospital organization is one of the key things here. The trustees have offered the physicians up to $100,000 to help set this up. . . . This money could go to hire a business manager for them who could then work with the hospital or negotiate with the hospital on some joint ventures that we may want to do through them.

McAuley, in recognition of the need to manage the overall change process, established a multiyear project funded equally by the health center, the medical staff, and the independent practice association for the purposes of envisioning and implementing a desired future state of practice in the coming decade. This is discussed in the concluding mini-case of this chapter.

Managing the Pace of Change

In dealing with hospital-physician relationships, it is particularly important that the pace of change be carefully managed. The key lies in knowing when to speed up the pace of change and when to slow it down. Effective executives were adept at knowing when to make decisions, create committees and ad hoc task forces, and use outside consultants and related means in order to quicken the pace of change and get people's attention. At the same time, they were sensitive to moments when change appeared to be occurring too rapidly. They were able to read the signs—increased physician tension, complaints, lack of communication, and things falling between the proverbial cracks. The need to accelerate the pace of change is indicated by the following comments of a McAuley executive:

> He [the CEO] wants to get some things off the dime, and he'll appoint special task forces or committees to do that. This organization doesn't react really well to that, but at the same time he [the CEO] is maybe trying to stimulate some things. . . . He kind of moves into the organization at times to get things really moving, then he'll back off in the end. If he sees the need for the organization to change, he believes firmly that if it is going to happen the person who is at the head of the organization needs to get in there and help do it. . . . Once it gets established, then I think he will pull back again.

An example of the need to slow down the pace of change is indicated by the following comments of a McAuley physician:

> It has been unusually difficult to get a third cath lab off the ground. A large part of that is financing. There are a lot of considerations involved and a lot of consensus seeking. Sometimes opportunities get advanced. . . . It is going very slowly but it is not terrible. . . . It is important that we not disrupt long-standing, supportive mutual relationships. Some people are young and impatient.

AN OVERALL MODEL

In reviewing the lessons and examples above, it is apparent that there are several elements involved in managing change, including the hospital's overall strategy, its structure, and its management processes. Strategic changes are usually long term and involve a major reorientation of an institution's plans (Shortell, Morrison, and Friedman 1990). Examples included North Monroe's desire to become a high-technology community medical center, Leonard Morse's desire to become a stronger force in managed care, Tucson Medical Center's interest in exploring regional merger relationships, and Sutter's intention to move from a horizontally integrated system to a more vertically integrated system featuring integrated medical campuses.

Changes in structure are usually of an intermediate time frame. They include determining the level at which key decisions are made, use of committees and task forces, and roles to be played by medical directors and related positions. Structure provides the forum in which change is implemented.

Process involves the short-term immediate day-to-day interactions among the key parties involved. It involves the micromanagement issues of daily communication, building and maintaining trust, and conflict management, described in earlier chapters.

These three elements are shown as overlapping circles in Figure 9.1. A key lesson of the study is the importance of aligning these elements as closely as possible. In brief, the greater the degree of overlap among these three elements the more successful were hospitals and physicians in initiating and implementing change. Structures (for example parallel organizations and ad hoc task forces) need to be established that are consistent with the organizational strategies (for example, vertical integration, managed care, focused diversification) and that facilitate timely, open, and accurate communication, collaborative problem solving, high-quality decision making, and trust. The looser the connections among strategy, structure, and process, the greater the problems in hospital-physician relationships. Takeuchi and Nonaka have likened the process to a rugby match versus a relay race (1986). Rather than sequential processing from strategy to structure to microprocesses (a relay race), a more effective approach is to have team members working back and forth among strategy, structure, and processes as they "move down the field" like a rugby team. Examples included McAuley's service line management approach, Tucson's service facilitator groups, and some of the activities of the physician-hospital organizations described in previous chapters.

Figure 9.1 Elements of Managing Change

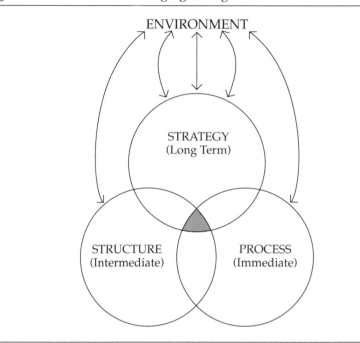

A factor in facilitating the overlap among the strategy, structure, and process elements was the stability of the key people involved. The stability of the top management team and key physician leaders enjoyed by almost all the study sites was a key factor in their success. Stability engendered trust. Trust engendered confidence in taking some risks and a willingness to experiment. Risk taking and experimentation, in turn, generated the opportunities for learning, and learning was an important reason for the success of many new initiatives. Frequent turnover of administration disrupts this cycle and the momentum gained, as reflected by numerous comments from North Monroe respondents, who during the period of the study lost their CEO. The comments of the following physician was typical of those made by most: "[Previous CEO] is one of the most honest and straightforward people you would want to meet. A real unique individual. I'm very anxious about the new person. I don't know much about him, but we need to be careful not to undo the good things that have happened here." The problems faced by the physicians that have frequent administrative turnover are well expressed by the following Leonard Morse physician: "There are changes every time we meet a new face. We go into the new administrators, the new faces, and we have to tell these people what has happened in the past. It's like starting all over again every time." In brief, stability is needed to manage change.

A second key ingredient in facilitating the overlap among strategy, structure, and process is the recognition on the part of hospital and physician leaders that they need to change themselves if they are to succeed in promoting organizational change. The desired change may require new attitudes, behaviors, skills, values, or some combination of these, as reflected in one physician's comments about his hospital's CEO:

> I think I see [CEO] and his staff listening more to what we are saying, being more responsive to our questions, and attending more meetings. I see a change in [CEO] at this period of time. I think that is very important. The [competing hospital] has an administrator who is an M.D. and who I think is tuned in to some of the changes. . . . But, I think that [hospital CEO] is the type of person who can make that change.

A MINICASE

On January 13, 1989, McAuley Health Center launched a major new initiative entitled PHYSICIANS 2000. This initiative serves as an example of an overall process of planned change. The project is sponsored jointly by the hospital's medical staff, the independent practice association of physicians (Huron Valley Physicians' Association), and the Catherine McAuley Health Center. Each group contributed an equal share of money to finance the three-year effort.

The purpose of PHYSICIANS 2000, in the words of a staff newsletter, is "to transform a local practice environment for physicians from one which is becoming increasingly influenced by negative factors into an environment which can be considered a magnet environment for retaining and attracting the most qualified and highly talented physicians." The specific objectives of PHYSICIANS 2000 are as follows:

1. to provide a forum in which the physician organizations and the Health Center can, together, plan for the future and address the many issues associated with change

2. to demonstrate to physicians the value of developing a vision of the future and of committing their time, energy, and resources to the achievement of these goals

3. to develop a consensus among physicians regarding a vision of the preferred practice environment to be achieved by the year 2000

4. to identify and support required planning and implementation activities

5. to involve as many physicians as possible in these endeavors

6. to communicate frequently to physicians about PHYSICIANS 2000 activities and national trends and developments

The opening retreat was attended by approximately 90 physicians and 30 members of the Health Center's administrative team. Based on the retreat, eight priority areas associated with a preferred practice environment were identified:

1. quality of care
2. the clinical practice environment
3. economic considerations
4. hospital-physician relationship
5. quality of life
6. malpractice issues
7. influence and recognition
8. relationships with the University of Michigan

Examples of specific objectives established for each area are indicated below:

Quality of Care

— The quality of care provided in all areas, ranging from acute inpatient to outpatient primary care to rehabilitative care will meet or exceed professional norms as well as criteria developed by consumers and purchasers of care.

— High-quality care will be maintained and enhanced through a process of continual improvement utilizing a variety of methods.

— Quality of care will be part of a total commitment by all types of providers to a continuous improvement process.

— The high quality achieved will result in the lowest malpractice rates in the Midwest, in provider-employer direct contracting, and in contracts with major payers at preferred rates.

Clinical Practice Environment

— Up-to-date, state-of-the-art technology will be provided consistent with the need to practice cost-effective medicine and consistent with the needs of patients in the primary and referral service areas.

— Physicians will have the necessary authority to make relevant patient care decisions.

— Continuing medical education programs will be of the highest quality and relevant to physician needs, interests, and the changing nature of the practice of medicine.

— Office practice operations will be more efficient and less costly.

Economic Issues

— A fair and equitable method of payment for different kinds of medical services will be operational and broadly supported by physicians.

— Practice management expenses will be efficiently managed.

— Income will be high enough to attract and retain high-quality physicians.

— Current patient volume will be maintained or increased.

— A dominant market position will be achieved and targeted in certain areas and market segments.

— Mutually beneficial, shared sponsorship arrangements for selected services will be developed.

Hospital-Physician Relationships

— A high level of trust and mutual respect will exist among all parties—physicians, other health professionals, and the hospital.

— An ongoing strategic planning process will involve all parties—physicians, other health professionals, and the hospital.

— Forums for managing honest disagreements and different responses to competitive conditions between and among physicians, other health professionals, and the hospital will be functioning effectively.

— A good balance of interest among different specialties, between hospital-based physicians and off-campus physicians, and between younger physicians and older physicians will be achieved.

Quality of Life

— Administrative and organizational mechanisms will be established that will permit physicians maximum time for providing patient care and engaging in relevant teaching and research.

— Professional and personal satisfaction will be enhanced by promoting the feeling of being part of a respected team—physicians, other health care professionals, and the hospital.

Malpractice

— A system that compensates claimants fairly and in a timely manner and that also takes into account the subtleties of the practice of medicine and provides some reasonable protection for physicians will be established.

— Malpractice insurance will be available to all types of physicians at reasonable and stable rates.

— Relationships between and among physicians, patients, and the hospital will become less adversarial.

Influence Processes

— Appropriate, time-effective ongoing relationships will be established with state legislators, major payers, and other relevant groups to promote ideas/actions consistent with the preferred future and to influence those ideas/actions that may be detrimental to the preferred future.

— Patients, regulators, legislators, payers, and public will have a better understanding and acceptance of the physician's role and work.

— Collaborative relationships will be developed with employers based on an understanding of their needs and on the provisions of services responsive to their needs.

— An ongoing relationship will be established with the University of Michigan for the purposes of continuing this discussion of mutual interests.

University of Michigan Relationships

— A relationship of mutual professional respect will be achieved.

— A forum for debating and resolving issues that cause conflict will be in place and functioning effectively.

— A plan to appropriately regionalize resources that draws on each institution's comparative advantages will have been developed and implemented.

— A system of integrated medical education between the two institutions will be in place.

During the first year, the PHYSICIANS 2000 steering committee composed of health center, IPA, and medical staff leaders met 16 times to discuss the overall agenda and specific issues. Greatest attention was given to the quality-of-care and clinical practice environment issues. In the area of quality of care, the PHYSICIANS 2000 project was responsible for adapting the health center's total quality initiative to physician needs. Specific accomplishments included

1. agreeing on the concept of total quality management training for physicians
2. defining the parameters of two courses
3. receiving approval from the medical staff executive committee
4. developing a subcommittee on course curriculum
5. arranging for an outside consultant to make a major presentation to the medical staff
6. obtaining continuing medical education credit for both courses
7. communicating to physicians about total quality management
8. informing physicians of educational opportunities through various medical staff and hospital newsletters

In the area of the clinical practice environment, the greatest attention was paid to recruitment and retention of primary care physicians and to the exploration of new practice models. In regard to recruitment and retention of primary care physicians, data were gathered from four primary care departments and individual physicians. A practice support committee was established, and several committees were formed to make recommendations. A key accomplishment has been the involvement of a large number of physicians in the definition of the issues and identification of solutions.

In regard to the exploration of alternative practice models, steering committee members and other physician leaders visited seven sites across the country to learn what others were doing. A variety of options were identified, ranging from loose networks of group practices to joint physician-hospital organizations to large multispecialty group practices. While most parties recognize that the current organization of physicians at McAuley is unlikely to be effective in the future, no clear picture of the preferred alternative arrangement has yet to be identified.

In addition to the above accomplishments, the project has invested considerable time and effort in communicating with all physicians on the staff. All parties involved believe that these efforts are beginning to pay off by raising the general level of awareness and knowledge about the issues confronting the practice of medicine in the area. Overall, an infrastructure has been created for ongoing communication and debate. The decision-making involvement of the three sponsoring groups has achieved closer integration. A common vision is beginning to emerge to provide overall direction to the different initiatives. More physicians have been energized to face the difficult issue of primary care physician recruitment and retention.

A vision statement of the preferred future has been developed to guide the project over the course of its existence:

> In our preferred future, the practice of medicine in the year 2000 will be characterized by high quality care which is driven by a process of continuous improvement which meets or exceeds professional, purchasers', and patients' criteria and which results in a high degree of professional and personal satisfaction and reasonable economic rewards. The ability to provide such care will take place within an environment of trust and mutual respect among physicians, other health professionals, and the hospital in which each party is given the means and sufficient autonomy to accomplish what they do best. The ability to provide such care will also take place within an environment in which each party individually and collectively can exert meaningful influence over external groups (for example, federal and state governments, major employers, the University of Michigan) who by their decisions can help promote or hinder preferred practice in this community.

GUIDELINES FOR MANAGING CHANGE

1. Diagnose what type of change is required—technical (means only), transitional (ends only), or transformational (change in both means and ends). Recognize that most issues involving hospitals and physicians are concerned with transformational change.

2. Use external and internal events to make people see the need for change. The status quo must be seen as personally uncomfortable, and the desire for change as an improvement in one's situation. At the same time, there is the need to be sensitive to a sense of loss and to allow a period of time for "grieving" over old practices, policies, and behavior.

3. Create a desired future state that appeals to personal, professional, and economic values and well-being.

4. Develop concrete, practical implementation steps that enable people to understand and buy into a process that will lead to the desired state.

5. Provide ongoing support and resources to make frequent adjustments as necessary.

6. Be sensitive to the pace of change, recognizing when things are moving too slowly and need to be speeded up, as well as when things are moving too fast and need to be slowed down.

7. Work with the above process to create an alignment or overlap among the hospital's long-run strategies, intermediate structures, and day-to-day processes so that they reinforce each other.

8. Create and maintain a perception of stability: "We are going to be here for the long run."

9. Recognize the need to change yourself and have the courage to do it.

REFERENCES

American Hospital Association. 1988. *The Emerging Roles of Physicians in Health Care Systems.* Section for Health Care Systems, Chicago, Il.

Gill, S. L., and S. S. Meighan. 1988. "Five Roadblocks to Effective Partnerships in a Competitive Health Care Environment," *Hospital and Health Services Administration* 33(Winter):505–20.

Kaluzny, A. D., and S. R. Hernandez. 1988. "Organizational Change and Innovation." In S. M. Shortell and A. D. Kaluzny (Eds.), *Healthcare Management: A Text in Organization Theory and Behavior.* 2nd ed., New York: John Wiley and Sons, 379–417.

Lewin, K. 1951. In D. Cartwright (Ed.), *Field Theory in Social Science.* New York: Harper and Row.

Shortell, S. M., E. M. Morrison, and B. Friedman. 1990. *Strategic Choices for America's Hospitals: Managing Change in Turbulent Times.* San Francisco: Jossey-Bass.

Takeuchi, H., and I. Nonaka. 1986. "The New Product Development Game," *Harvard Business Review* (January-February):137–46.

PART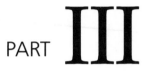

Special Issues

CHAPTER 10

Hospital-Physician Competition

Prior to the 1980s, hospitals and physicians were seldom in direct competition with each other. Conflicts primarily centered around the speed with which the hospital could purchase new technology and expand existing facilities and services; differences within the medical staff involving issues of privileging and credentialing; and, in some cases, personality differences between CEOs and key physician leaders. With the advent of prospective payment and related initiatives designed to contain hospital costs, conflicting incentives were established for hospitals and physicians. Further, many hospitals saw the need to diversify by developing new programs and services. It was expected that these services would both generate increased referrals to the hospital and additional revenue in their own right. These activities were perceived by some physicians as direct competition. Examples included hospital efforts to develop satellite primary care centers, ambulatory surgery centers, and urgent care centers. Other physicians, not directly threatened by the loss of patients, were philosophically opposed to those activities as constituting the "corporate practice of medicine." Specialists were often opposed on the grounds that the resources being spent on such programs could be better used in developing inpatient "centers of excellence." Hospitals did not help their cause when many of the new ventures were developed with little or no physician input, where physician input was ignored, or where the new ventures proved to be unprofitable (Shortell, Wickizer, and Wheeler 1984).

Until recently, most of the competition was unidirectional, that is, the hospital competing with physicians. In recent years, the competition has become increasingly bidirectional (National Health Policy Forum 1989). Physicians are now competing with hospitals in developing new programs and services, particularly in regard to ancillary testing and treatment involving laboratory, radiology, and pharmaceutical services. Given the continued growth of managed care, featuring discounted payment and congressional approval of a relative value–based fee schedule linked to overall physician expenditure targets, the economic environment for physicians will become even more stringent. It may not be long before the economic pressures facing physicians are similar in severity and magnitude to those facing hospitals (Estes Park Institute 1990). The net result is an environment that can lead to increased competition between the two groups.

STUDY SITES' EXPERIENCES

For the most part, the ten sites did well in managing hospital-physician competition. There was little or no competition at six sites and low to moderate at the remaining four. In no site was there a high degree of competition. These judgments are supported by questionnaire data. For example, the hospital-physician competition scale received an overall mean rating of 3.81 (1 to 5 scale, where 1 = low satisfaction and 5 = high satisfaction), with a range from 3.5 to 4.4. A closely related scale measuring physician recruitment also received a relatively high evaluation of 3.78, with a range from 3.2 to 4.2.

There are several approaches that the study sites used to manage competitive issues:

1. advanced planning and extensive consultation including a strong role played by medical staff leadership
2. developing new organizational forms (for example, joint physician-hospital organizations and joint venture arrangements) to address competitive issues
3. using the outside environment to encourage cooperative rather than competitive relationships
4. not overreacting to physician competitive initiatives

Advanced Planning and Consultation

Several of the sites—Crouse-Irving Memorial, Lexington, and Sutter— learned from early experience the importance of involving physicians in the hospital's plans to pursue ambulatory care diversification initiatives. Each of the three sites ran into some problems from moving too quickly and from being perceived as not sufficiently involving some physicians in the planning activities. At the same time, other sites such as Leonard Morse and McAuley adopted policies of always consulting physicians on their diversification plans and choosing not to go ahead if physicians failed to support the idea. As a result, some opportunities were lost. The hospitals, however, were willing to make this trade-off in order to build stronger long-run relationships. Scripps followed a similar policy but admitted that, given the increasingly competitive environment in its area, it might choose to go ahead with some programs in the future even if physicians disagreed. It added that this would be done very cautiously. In general, the hospital-physician competition issues were greatest for those sites facing the most competition in their external environment.

The above issues and approaches are reflected in the following set of comments. From a Lexington physician:

> We [the hospital] built an urgent care center. [CEO name] offered it to the family practitioners, but they said no. Then the hospital went ahead anyway, and it's losing money. They tried to ram a square peg into a round hole. . . . Our medical staff leadership at times had had to step in and put out the fire.

At McAuley a medical staff–appointed committee is used to deal with competitive issues. As explained by a McAuley executive:

> There is a physician committee appointed by the chief of staff that reviews all projects to assess competition both between the hospital and physicians and among the physicians before any project goes forward. . . . There are some things that have really been slowed down because of that. So, ironically, some of the physicians may step out and start competing with the hospital through joint ventures . . . going around the other side. . . . For example, there was a prostate screening clinic that took a year and a half to get through this process. Had the medical executive committee not approved it the other night, the urologist would have done it privately.

The situation involving an ambulatory care satellite was described by a board member at Crouse-Irving Memorial:

> The satellite center issue reached me as an individual board member. But it has not been discussed at a board meeting. One physician mentioned to me that they weren't given sufficient chance to be involved in that endeavor. I mentioned it to our medical director, and he indicated that they had sufficient notice. It was in the minutes of the meetings that were discussed and in the marketing committee minutes. Some of these physicians maybe weren't in attendance or didn't read the minutes. They should have known. It

may be an issue with a few physicians, but I don't think it's a serious issue. . . . I think the physician's complaint was that the old guard and the people that were department heads had first crack, and all the others didn't seem to be included in the window of communication. That was his complaint.

At the same time, the following comments of a Crouse-Irving Memorial physician indicate the importance of multiple forms of communication (see Chapter 6):

I guess it was generally announced at the executive committee meeting. Those minutes go out to the medical staff, but we know they don't read anything that comes to them anyway. So they obviously didn't see it. I personally don't think it was widespread. I don't think the announcement about what we wanted to do was fairly distributed to our physicians so that they could then apply or demonstrate an interest. After that, there still would have to be a selection process if there were too many interested. But I think the big problem now is that physicians don't feel that they were even informed of the possibility. So I think that if we did anything like that again, I would hope that we would have much better communication.

The spirit of cooperation at Tucson Medical Center is captured in the following physician's words:

The hospital has been very cooperative. But, you know, you can't help but do that. . . . The hospital has gone out of their way to insure that the majority, probably not all, but the majority of physicians on the staff are aware of what's being done and feel that it's in the best interest of everybody.

The following comments of a board member at North Monroe reflect the extent to which positive physician attitudes can foster a cooperative spirit:

Why change a good thing? We're going to keep doing what we're doing. For instance, my doctor is [doctor's name], a very fine nephrology man and internist. There are three in his clinic. He's got a lot of people on the kidney dialysis machine here and treats them here at this hospital. He told me that to check my heart out he had to do an EKG and that he could do it on me in his office or at the hospital. And I said, "Well, you want to do all of this at your clinic because you make more money that way, or do you want me to go out to the hospital?" I also needed a stress test. He said that they do the best deal at the hospital on some of the tests and on others he said he could do some of it in the clinic. So he referred me to the hospital for most of my work. And that's a prime example of a situation where the doctor absolutely isn't holding back anything as far as competitiveness is concerned.

In response to possible future competition, a North Monroe executive expressed the hospital's approach:

In regard to future competition, we would probably try to come up with some alternatives and look at the problem. Off the top of my head, I can think of several alternatives. We could either offer a joint venture to them, or we could give them a share of what we are doing over at the clinic, depending on how serious they were. More than likely they wouldn't do that because they realize that would make the hospital mad and severely impact the relationship between the clinic and the hospital. That's something that everyone is trying to maintain. If it [competition] did occur, we could try the joint venturing approach. . . . If that didn't work, more than likely we would look at whether the benefits outweigh the costs. How much revenue are we going to lose from the deal compared to how much revenue they put into the hospital? Now if they're putting $5 million revenue a year and I'm going to lose $200,000, it wouldn't be worth fighting over. Now if the situation were reversed and we're going to lose $3 million and they've put in only $2.5 million revenue, then we'd have to look at it with a little stronger approach. I have no idea what we'd do, but we'd definitely come up with something. More likely we would try to maintain a positive relationship.

A somewhat contrasting view is offered by a Providence physician:

The crazy thing about it is that physicians expect to compete with the hospital. They don't think a thing about it to open an ambulatory surgery center next door or down the hill. But if the hospital opens a clinic down the hill, oh, my God! That's raping your sister. That doesn't count. I think that's an area where [the CEO] should say, you're competing with me and you say I can't compete with you. . . . The hospital has opened some primary care clinics, but they're all out in the suburbs where they don't really compete with the staff. I think they ought to compete with the staff. I think competition's healthy. I think it makes us all better.

Despite the various approaches described above, all agreed that the intensity of competition between the two will grow in the future. As expressed by a McAuley executive:

> We have a situation with a prostate program. We're trying to look at ways that we can move forward together in a win-win situation. We've spent a lot of time trying to determine how to do that kind of thing. We've had a couple of physicians who have wanted to have their cake and eat it, too. They wanted to have their own ultrasound in their office but also wanted to participate in the clinic. The agreement had been that if you participate in the clinic, you're going to get the referrals, and as a result you don't need to compete with the radiologists from the hospital. The medical staff said we needed to respect what it was, and we agreed on it. . . . So the competition issue, I think, is heating up. The cardiologists are now saying that they want to renegotiate their exclusive contract because maybe they can do better. So there is some of that occurring, and it's on the uprise.

Alternative Organizational Forms

Alternative organizational forms such as physician-hospital organizations (PHOs) and joint venture arrangements were frequently used to channel potential conflicting situations. The role played by the PHO is described by a Tucson executive as follows:

> One of the agreements of the PHOs is that if there's something we're not currently doing, before we consider doing it we'll go to the physicians and say, do you want to joint venture with us? It's sort of the right of first refusal on emerging opportunities.

This experience is further elaborated by a second Tucson executive:

> Basically, what we try to do in terms of competition is indicated by a situation that we had with our radiologists. They decided they wanted to establish an imaging center and sell shares in it to the doctors. A lot of doctors thought that was a great idea. There had been an imaging center developed over at [name of hospital] by some doctors and limited shares were sold. Some doctors made pretty good money on it. I had lunch one day with one of the physicians and said that I was concerned with what I heard was going on between Radiology Limited and SAIP [Southern Arizona Independent Physicians] because what this represented is that Radiology Limited was going to go into the CT business, which had been kept in the hospital up to that point in time. So I said, "I'm

really concerned about this." I said, "I'm even more concerned because it seems to me that this is specifically the kind of thing that we said the PHO would be used for, at least as a focus for discussion." He said, "God, you're right." We brought it into the PHO and, basically, constructed a deal where TMC [Tucson Medical Center] would have a piece of if, the PHO would have a piece of it, individual physicians would have a piece of it, and we were creating something that we thought was going to be a win-win-win situation. Then the lawyers got involved with multiple antitrust concerns, and we're still working it out. . . . But a potentially serious divisive thing was really defused using the PHO. We are also using the PHO to implement our satellite care center strategy, which is directed at preventing it from being a hospital-physician competition issue. And it's interesting. I think the projects have been better by virtue of the fact that they've been joint hospital-physician projects.

Sutter's experience in working with joint ventures is highlighted by the following executive's comments:

We've had a lot of developments with our radiologists. They were trying to put an imaging center joint venture together with us, and at the same time we had separate negotiations going on over clinical services. The president of the radiology group would call me and try to trade one off for the other. I'd say, "I'm sorry [doctor's name], but you know they're two different issues." . . . As I've said to our management team, "Hey, you've got to understand why they're [the physicians] doing it. They're frightened that they're losing income sources. They're diversifying in their own way just like we are." So our approach has been to try to work with them where we can. . . . Because of some of our joint ventures, we are doing 50 percent more surgeries than we would have done before.

The important role played by the XIMED physician organization at Scripps is described below by one of the organization's physicians:

We have tried to present ourselves in an organized manner to use our organizational structures as the primary method for communicating with the hospital. Time and time again we've told our people not to fragment. Don't go off with your special projects. Make sure you run it through the medical staff or XIMED. We try to keep a reliable, consistent organization that the administration can deal with and that we can deal with. We feel this is probably the most important thing we can do.

Using the Outside Environment

As discussed in Chapter 9, effective executives used the outside environmental pressures to encourage needed change. These same forces (managed care, increased external competition, etc.) were also used to encourage joint hospital-physician undertakings and to avoid competing with each other. This was particularly true in regard to managed care (see the next chapter). As expressed by a West Allis executive: "We want contracts that will benefit both of us. We want to make sound business decisions that will benefit both." A McAuley physician expressed the same sentiment by noting: "It is important that physicians get together with their hospital. You need to present a united front, or they will pick you off."

The Importance of Not Overreacting

As previously noted, physicians were increasingly competing with hospitals by doing more radiology, laboratory, and related ancillary services in their offices and clinics. Most of the hospitals felt it important not to overreact to these developments. They tried to understand the situation from the physician's perspective (for example, see the Sutter executive's previously cited comments). If the physician could perform the procedure as well as the hospital, the hospital essentially "looked the other way and bit their tongue." They had matured to understanding the relationship from a business perspective. The following situations are illustrative.

A Leonard Morse board member described a situation involving a group of orthopedists as follows:

> Last year a couple of orthopedists put an x-ray unit in their office building. I think their radiologists were more upset than we were and asked us to go to battle for them. We felt the orthopedists were more important and that it wasn't going to be that big of an issue. We let them do that. We'd rather keep them happy and maintain the patients. The way the reimbursement system works in Massachusetts right now is that the inpatient stay is much more profitable than the outpatient business. . . . So although you do make some dollars on the outpatient side, I would rather not alienate a physician that's giving us the inpatient volume or who would be willing to do so if they wanted to do some more of the outpatient work in their office. What I understand from the physician reimbursement side is that coming in to the hospital for them is not terribly lucrative anymore.

A Scripps executive describes a sports medicine venture in the following words:

> We have had some services in which physicians were sucking business away. . . . Sports medicine is a good example of that. The orthopods saw the volume building up and decided they would go off and start one of their own. . . . It hurts, I've got to admit it. We weren't really pleased when it happened because we just bought the business. . . . I think we realized that it was a business decision. We just wish they would have been more up front about it before we had bought it. . . . Another example is the ophthalmologists. We've got one who used to be very supportive of our efforts in this area and then threatened to take is all back in his office. We responded to that by compromising, forming a practice corporation and leasing him the equipment. We're hurt financially but not as bad as if he'd done it all on his own. We can't blame him. The government is really giving them incentives to move it out of the hospital.
>
> Another case in point involved a women's center where we wanted to staff an office and make it available on a rotating basis for physicians that wanted to use it. The medical staff was very opposed to that, and they ultimately prevailed. We wanted to do it as a strategic imperative. We said, "OK, we'll back off and develop a different model that won't be as threatening to you. We don't want to go to war about this." Another example is occupational medicine. We thought we [the hospital] could play a big role in that. But we sensed that our primary care physicians felt so intimidated that it would be too much competition so we backed away from it. We are trying to find a way in which we might be able to work together. That's currently under discussion.

The same Scripps executive also described how they might deal with these issues in the future:

> If it's something we sense that's going to be competitive, we'll try to work out a way that we might do it together. I think that's more true now than it was maybe two years ago. But let's say for sake of discussion that it wasn't going to work for one reason or another, and we still felt it was strategically important for the hospital to go ahead. I think we'd be tempted to move ahead. We'd like their comments. If there are still strong objections to it, I suppose at that point we'd stop and take a second look at it. We might or might not go forward. . . . I think philosophically we both understand there are areas where we may disagree and we'll both work to minimize

those areas, and there may be some places where we'll still have to
be competitive. I think they've gotten to a point where they understand that. They told me that. There will be deals that we'll do that
they won't like and vice versa, but our point is to try and make sure
they understand why we're doing it. At this point in the relationship, we share more than they do. We understand that we
operate in a fishbowl and that even if we wanted to keep something secret, it couldn't be. Some of their top leadership still
doesn't know that they deal in a fishbowl, and I'll find out things
that they're talking about as if they're trying to keep it from me. It
just doesn't work, but they'll learn that over time. That's just a
maturing process. We all understand that our futures are dependent on each other's success. We have the dialogue and the trust is
growing. I think we'll be successful together.

It is also of interest to note that the Scripps board has a written policy
supporting the private practice of medicine. This is viewed by the physicians as a very important substantive, as well as symbolic, gesture of
goodwill on the hospital's part. In the same vein as the comment of the
Scripps executive, a West Allis executive noted:

Our anesthesiologist group was actually soliciting our surgeons to
start a separate ambulatory surgery center. We had to step in. We
told them it was us or them. They backed off. . . . It's important to
not overreact, but you also have to be firm. Overall, we tend not to
get too excited about things. . . . We try to let the doctors decide
what they want to do, and then we try to help finance it and work
with it.

CONCLUDING OBSERVATIONS

Economic, social, and technological forces will lead to an increasingly
challenging relationship for hospitals and physicians. These forces will
present opportunities for *both* collaboration and competition. If the experience of the ten sites is any guide, the key to success will be the ability
of hospitals and physicians to work together as economic business partners to complement their ability to work together as clinical partners.
This will require both groups to recognize the legitimacy, and indeed
necessity, of making decisions on good business criteria after assuring
that clinical criteria are met. Both groups need to learn that saying no to
each other at times and going one's own way is OK. It can be done
without losing respect or trust. The key lies in how each party conducts

themselves in the negotiations and discussions. The transformation of the American health care system demands a corresponding transformation of its infrastructure—the heart of which is the hospital-physician relationship. Some guidelines for moving along this pathway of maturity and transformation are summarized below.

GUIDELINES AND BEST PRACTICES FOR MANAGING COMPETITION

1. Wherever possible, hospitals and physicians should discuss new business opportunities with each other first. These opportunities should be evaluated for both their short-run and long-run implications, taking into account economic, clinical, and service criteria.

2. Organizational mechanisms should be developed to serve as forums for such discussions. These may range from joint committees to economic joint venture corporations to joint physician-hospital organizations. It is important that both groups understand and feel comfortable with the mechanisms established for reviewing joint opportunities.

3. It is important that both hospitals and physicians not overreact when decisions are made that are perceived to be against their interests. As discussed in Chapter 8 in managing conflict, both groups need to recognize that they will have to live with each other in the long run. Thus, it is important that the relationship not be severely damaged as a result of a decision perceived negatively by one group.

4. The greater the extent to which issues can be anticipated during the institution's strategic planning process with heavy physician involvement, the more likely it is that the issue will receive appropriate discussion, and unnecessary conflict and competitiveness will be forestalled.

5. Continued programs of physician leadership education and involvement are important for appropriate and relevant physician input so as to keep the competitive situations in appropriate context.

REFERENCES

Estes Park Institute Conference. 1990. "Marketplace Warfare: Hospitals and Physicians in Competitive Environments," Kona, Hawaii, January 16–20.

National Health Policy Forum. 1989. "Competitive Struggles Between Hospitals and Physicians: The Federal Angle," Issue Brief #525, George Washington University, Washington, DC, July 27.

Shortell, S. M., T. M. Wickizer, and J. R. C. Wheeler, Jr. 1984. *Hospital-Physician Joint Ventures: Results and Lessons from a National Demonstration.* Ann Arbor, MI: Health Administration Press.

CHAPTER 11

Managed Care

Dealing with managed care was one of the most frequently mentioned issues placing stress on the hospital-physician relationship at nearly all sites. In a few sites, over 70 percent of inpatient hospital revenues were derived from managed care payment sources. As expressed by a West Allis physician:

> Managed care is the issue. I really think both the hospital and the doctors are trying to do the job in spite of managed care. This would be the best way I can put it. Managed care can get in the way. We do all the things we ever did for people—order all the same tests, do all the same procedures, and spend the same amount of time with people. In addition, we deal with the managed care system. The managed care system is superimposed on what we're doing, and from our view it doesn't make anything efficient at all. It's just another factor to cope with. And a whole new, vast population of people that are living off of health care are now getting in the way.

On average, most of the sites studied felt that they were dealing with managed care in an appropriate fashion, as indicated by a satisfaction level of 3.8 (1-low to 5-high). Nonetheless, there was considerable variation, with a range of 2.5 to 4.3. The experience of each of the sites is briefly highlighted below followed by a set of conclusions and guidelines for managing relationships in the future.

TEN SITES' EXPERIENCES

Crouse-Irving Memorial Hospital

For the most part, managed care issues were not salient at Crouse-Irving Memorial Hospital. Stringently enforced health-planning legislation in the 1970s and 1980s reduced the number of hospitals in the Syracuse area from nine to four. This resulted in a relatively efficient delivery system and little impetus for HMO, PPO, or related alternative delivery system approaches. As a result, the major employers in the area have not yet been vocal in demanding more cost-effective approaches to care.

Leonard Morse Hospital

Leonard Morse had a negative experience with an HMO in the early 1980s. The physicians who joined the plan felt that the hospital derived greater financial benefits than the physicians. The plan lost money and eventually folded. As a result, the hospital has had problems getting its physicians, particularly specialists, to try again. Many of the physicians' practices remain full, so there are few incentives to join alternative plans. Nonetheless, about one-quarter of the staff is involved in some managed care activity, primarily in behavioral medicine. The hospital's board has played an important role in getting the physicians to stay involved. The hospital has formed a joint physician-hospital organization to investigate further managed care involvement. This is strategically important for Leonard Morse because many of its competing hospitals have significant involvement in managed care activities.

Lexington Medical Center

Lexington Medical Center and its physicians have also had differences in their views towards HMOs. The hospital turned down one HMO that the physicians had joined because the hospital did not want to give discounts, angering the physicians involved. The hospital has now softened its stance somewhat and has begun some HMO discounting. The hospital and the physicians are now thinking about developing their own managed care plan with the intention of marketing it directly to industry.

McAuley Health Center

Like Leonard Morse, McAuley Health Center had an early negative experience with HMO involvement, but for a different reason. McAuley and members of its medical staff (organized as Huron Valley Physicians' Association, an IPA) felt that they had jointly developed their own HMO in the Ann Arbor area. Mercy Health Services (of which McAuley is a member), however, claimed ultimate ownership rights and control over the HMO. The corporate office centralized administrative control over the plan, leaving the local McAuley physicians embittered. This decision and its subsequent consequences have had a marked impact on the relationship between McAuley Health Center's administration and its physicians. As expressed by one McAuley physician:

> The feeling on the part of some of the medical staff is that that plan was ours and we made it succeed and then they [the corporate office] took it away from us. That's the perception. As a result of that, how they now deal with that health plan and everything associated with it is much different. . . . I think the feeling was that this hospital [McAuley] might carry weight, have more clout when it came to these kinds of things than it really did. Not that the hospital couldn't carry a lot of clout and that a lot of things occurred in the past because of the success of this place and because of the caliber of our administration. But you push it to the limit at that particular point, it didn't turn out the way it was anticipated. . . . I don't know whether they saw it coming or not. . . . The administration, though, tried not to let their disappointment show, and I'm sure their anger and other kinds of things kind of ruled the day. But if they had been angry and expressed it openly, it just would have led to the medical staff being more angry and frustrated and all of those other things. So it's really more a matter of degree than anything else. But I think the tempering of that was very important. . . . They [the administration] don't necessarily agree with it. But I guess the word is acceptance.

While a number of McAuley physicians continue to stay involved with the local plan (as operated by the corporate office), significant dissatisfaction remains. There is a possibility that some aspects of the plan's administration may once again be decentralized. In the meantime, a number of lessons have been learned:

1. the need to recognize that managed care is a business
2. the need to develop strong information systems to track utilization and costs
3. the need to watch over your own budget
4. the need to develop a sound business plan

The physicians also believe it's extremely important to present a united front with the hospital or "third party payers will pick you off."

North Monroe Hospital

There is no managed care activity at North Monroe. This reflects the hospital's location in Louisiana, where alternative forms of medical practice have not yet taken root. Nonetheless, the hospital is potentially positioning itself for such development through its encouragement of the Northern Louisiana Medical Clinic, whose physicians practice almost exclusively at the hospital.

Providence Medical Center

Providence has had a generally positive experience in dealing with managed care. In large part, this is due to the development of a network of primary care satellites in the late 1970s and early 1980s. This network has given them leverage in negotiating contracts. It has been particularly helpful in dealing with multispecialty groups on the medical staff. In essence, the primary care satellite can say to the specialist, "You need to sign these contracts that we're getting involved in if you want to get the referrals from us."

Scripps Memorial Hospital

Scripps operates in a highly competitive HMO managed care environment. It is involved in approximately 40 HMO/PPO contracts, representing about 25 percent of their revenues. The primary vehicle on the physicians' part for negotiating these contracts is the XIMED physician organization. Because the hospital and the physicians do not negotiate as a single entity with outside peers, the potential exists for disagreements over particular contracts in which either the hospital or the physicians want to go ahead but not the other party. This occurred when Aetna radically changed its contract with XIMED, resulting in cancellation. This caused considerable concern on the part of the hospital and selected physicians. Some felt it would be the first significant test of physicians' loyalty to XIMED.

Sutter Health

Like Scripps, Sutter faces considerable managed care competition. Unlike Scripps, however, the primary competition is from one source, Kaiser, which has about 32 percent of the inpatient market in the Sacramento area. Sutter has chosen to battle Kaiser head-to-head. Two large groups of physicians have formed—the Capitol Medical Group and the Sacramento Sierra Medical Group. Between them, these two groups of physicians, who practice primarily at Sutter Community Hospitals, have approximately 180,000 enrollees versus 400,000 for Kaiser. The presence of the groups has enabled them to negotiate more favorable managed care contracts than the individual providers could arrange for themselves. Sutter devotes considerable effort to strengthening these two groups. Among the possibilities include a merger of the two groups to be the exclusive provider for Foundation Health, Inc. (an HMO partially owned by Sutter), which would enable them to compete more strongly against Kaiser. Sutter's philosophy is "Future health care business will not be won simply by providing better care or by cultivating patient relationships. The provider organization with the best marketing position in the trade area wins." Toward this end, the Sutter board and physician leadership has agreed to the following objectives:

1. Develop a unified third party payer plan.
2. Create a variety of hospital-physician relationship options, from support of solo fee-for-service medicine through IPA/PPO arrangements to group practice and HMO panel participation opportunities.
3. Enhance physician loyalty; build trust.
4. Create economic incentives so that members of the medical staff will not support competitors' products.
5. Establish relationships between the hospital and physicians that foster mutual support and discourage competitive product development.
6. Create a larger and more pluralistic value-added health distribution system than Kaiser Permanente.
7. Assure the best tertiary care in Sacramento.

A full-time executive is employed to implement these objectives and oversee all managed care contracting.

Tucson Medical Center

Like Scripps and Sutter, Tucson Medical Center (TMC) is in a market characterized by intense competition between physicians and hospitals for managed care contracts. In addition, physicians in Tucson have relatively little loyalty to any particular hospital. In the past, TMC lost two major contracts and came to realize that they could not just be a contractor in the managed care business but needed to form their own managed care vehicle. The initial response was the formation of a PPO open to all TMC staff. Later, a small group of independent physicians known as the Southern Arizona Independent Physicians (SAIP) joined with TMC in forming a joint physician-hospital organization. One of its main objectives is to bind a core group of physicians closer to the hospital and to generate more loyalty and mutual dependence. It has an advisory board, comprised of eight members from two parent organizations, with equal representation from the hospital and the physician side. It has also become the vehicle for administration of a managed health care plan. TMC specialists have been slow in recognizing HMO activities, particularly in regard to the emerging importance of the primary care physician. TMC, however, feels that progress is being made. As described by one executive:

> I think our doctors really have bought into a view of the future that's going to be a managed care future. You can "game" the system in the short term, but the only way you're going to succeed in the long term is to play the managed care game and grab a large enough share of the market, and at a reduced rate of utilization you can still make it up in volume. . . . When we decided to form the HMO, we suggested that we share it with them half and half. And they said, "Well, you know, how much is that going to cost?" And we told them how much. And then they said, "Well, you know, that's not a very good investment. That's a lot of money." And we said, "We understand that." We feel that if we're going to be successful as an HMO, if we're going to differentiate ourselves by being the HMO where the physicians have an equal say with the hospitals, then we should do it. So we gave them a split in governance even with no financial investment. And that was not easy to sell within our own management group or with our boards. Some of our board members, you know, are capitalists with a capital C, and they just could not fathom giving someone a 50 percent say in something if they don't have a 50 percent investment. But we've been able to convince them of that. And when our physicians go talk to other physicians about what we're doing, they'll say, "You know, the difference in our system is we have as much say as the hospital about what that damned thing is going to do and we don't have a nickel invested. All we've got is our commitment to it and our time involved. And they use that as a selling point with their peers." I think that helped them develop that feeling of trust with us.

The lack of shared financial risk flies in the face of recommended practice, but TMC believes it is necessary as an initial step in order to secure needed physician involvement. As in several of the other sites, the biggest threat to the HMO relationship at Tucson is the subspecialists' concerns over the increased role of primary care.

West Allis Memorial

In 1983, West Allis was the first hospital in Wisconsin to attempt to start a PPO. It failed because, in their words, "we really didn't know what we were doing." Since then, the hospital has had a number of encounters with HMOs. In one case, the CEO encouraged physicians to re-sign an HMO contract even though the hospital would lose $1 million in revenue. Most of the physicians followed the CEO's advice. The board supported the CEO's decision. In a second case, the CEO encouraged physicians to sign an HMO contract, but the physicians decided it was not in their best interest. In both cases, economic circumstances drove the decision and both parties understood the criteria being used and respected each other's wishes.

The hospital has an IPA to negotiate contracts. They try to use the profits from either the hospital or the physician to subsidize the other part as needed. The CEO sits on the board of the IPA and the executive committee so they can plan together. As the CEO notes, "we want contracts that will benefit both of us." Overall, there is a 30 percent penetration rate of managed care providers in West Allis's market.

SUMMARY OBSERVATIONS

Based on the brief highlights of the above experiences, several observations may be made. First, it is important for the hospital and physicians to present a united front to third parties. Without presenting a united front, there is the potential for the agreement to be more favorable for one party than the other. If it is not possible to present a united front in all cases (for example, Lexington, Scripps, West Allis), some of the sites are experimenting with approaches in which the party that does better financially helps to subsidize the other party (for example, West Allis). This, of course, depends on having established a strong level of trust between the parties involved.

Second, involvement in managed care forces both hospitals and physicians to reexamine the kinds of physicians that they want involved. From the hospital's perspective, the main interest is in bonding the most loyal physicians to the institution. From both the hospital's and physicians' perspective, the economic incentives are to involve those physicians that practice the most cost-effective medicine. Thus, the sites are coming to realize the need for stringent credentialing and utilization review. This was perhaps most pronounced at Tucson Medical Center. This often results in a subgroup of physicians who participate in the arrangement, which, in turn, can lead to inevitable political battles. In order to deal with these conflicts, it is necessary for strong physician leadership to exert its influence, as expressed by a Tucson Medical Center executive:

> In managed care, they [the physicians] got to have some control over their people. So they don't want more physicians than they

need to provide the services or more physicians than they can control because utilization review is very important. So they need to judge how many orthopedic surgeons they need, where they are located, and so on. The other criteria [sic] is . . . are they good people? Also, do they practice cost-effectively? Are they going to behave responsibly from an economic standpoint? And another, quite frankly, is TMC loyalty. You have to have a combination of all those things or we won't let you in.

Third, managed care is forcing younger physicians to practice more in groups. To the extent that this trend continues, it may make it somewhat easier for hospitals and physicians to select those groups of physicians that might be most appropriate for managed care relationships. At the same time, it can present problems where groups of specialists or primary care physicians are in strong competition with each other. Nonetheless, in the words of one administrator, "It is much easier to herd clusters of cats than it is to herd a bunch of individual strays."

Finally, the experiences of the ten sites demonstrate the importance of hospitals and physicians maturing in their relationship as business partners. At every site, each party was beginning to recognize the legitimate economic interests of the other. Each understood why a given contract might be more or less beneficial to the other and that the benefits would not necessarily be congruent with each other. While each recognized the advantages of presenting a united front where possible, they also recognized that at times one of them might need to sign a contract that would not be in the best interests of the other. Each, however, recognized that in the long run the economic interests of both needed to be met and, therefore, some transfer payment arrangements or related mechanisms needed to be considered.

GUIDELINES FOR DEVELOPING MORE EFFECTIVE MANAGED CARE RELATIONSHIPS

The experiences of the study sites suggest the following major guidelines. These are consistent with those documented in a recent study of four major HMOs (Fox and Heinen 1987).

1. There is a need to select high-quality physicians who are cost-effective providers. Mechanisms must be designed in advance to select such physicians, or rigorous review systems instituted that can select out such providers after appropriate experience under the plan.

2. Physician involvement in the management of the plan is important. Physician executives, such as the medical director, can play a key role in confronting colleagues on such issues as utilization.

3. There is a need for continuous education regarding the importance of practicing cost-effective medicine. Physicians must be made aware of the impact of high utilization and the relationship between efficient medical care and the quality of care.

4. There is need to establish an organizational vehicle (for example, an PHO or related mechanism) that provides a forum for both the hospital and physicians to consider managed care options.

5. Wherever possible, a united front must be presented to third-party purchasers.

6. There is the need to recognize that managed care is a business.

7. The importance of primary care physicians to the economic and professional success of specialists must be demonstrated.

8. There must be ongoing responsiveness to physician concerns.

REFERENCE

Fox, P. D., and L. Heinen. 1987. *Determinants of HMO Success.* Ann Arbor, MI: Health Administration Press.

CHAPTER 12

Hospital-Physician Joint Ventures

One way in which hospitals and physicians have responded to the forces facing them has been through the development of economic joint ventures. An economic joint venture is an arrangement to provide services in which each party is at financial risk and stands to gain a financial reward. Examples include HMO or PPO development, technology acquisition, building and leasing of medical office buildings, establishing ambulatory surgery centers or diagnostic testing centers, and providing nonhealth lines of business such as real estate. Joint ventures can have potential benefits by enabling each party to obtain needed capital that neither could obtain alone, sharing financial risk, facilitating hospital-physician communication and involvement in joint decision making, insuring cost-effective use of resources, and helping to avoid conflict-of-interest issues and, sometimes, certificate-of-need requirements (Coopers and Lybrand 1988). Potential disadvantages include antitrust and inurement risks, issues associated with exclusivity, the danger of one party failing to fulfill their obligations, and the loss of control and flexibility that comes from each party being able to act on their own initiative.

Among the study sites, McAuley, Scripps, Sutter, and Tucson Medical Center had the most involvement in joint venture activities; Crouse-Irving Memorial, Leonard Morse, Providence, and West Allis had some experience; and Lexington and North Monroe, little or no involvement. The experience of each of the sites is highlighted below.

TEN SITES' EXPERIENCES

McAuley Health Center

McAuley had some early joint venture experience in providing facilities and staff for cardiology and gastroenterology services. The profits from these efforts were shared between the hospital and the physicians. The ventures were eventually dissolved due to Blue Cross's and Medicare's refusal to pay facility fees and difficulties of communication between the physician groups and the hospital.

More recent joint venture activities have included a successful physician office building and a less successful HMO, previously described in Chapter 11. One of the hospital's physician executives believes that the negative HMO experience has facilitated their learning, commenting that "we looked at it as a family enterprise instead of as a hard business deal." The hospital and its physicians have now formed Allegiance Corporation, a joint physician-hospital organization, to serve as a vehicle for future joint ventures and HMO involvement. Their past experience suggests that the less successful ventures suffered primarily from poor communication, lack of common expectations, or both. They found these issues to be particularly prominent when trying to deal with two specialty groups in competition with each other. One example is expressed in the following comments of a McAuley executive:

> Right now we're trying to deal with it on a departmental basis. . . . We have a fairly hot issue right now with a prostate screening clinic. We have said to the department of urology that we'd like to have all members of the department involved. . . . That has been difficult to put into place because you have . . . two major practices that compete like hell with each other. The two principals used to be in practice together and then split apart. They both have very high quality people with very large practices—about four or five men in each of the two groups. They compete like crazy. So we try to get them to work together, but it is very difficult. We're trying to avoid picking one group versus another as being principal partner on the venture.

Another issue faced by McAuley and the other sites is exclusivity, that is, the extent to which the joint venture opportunities are open to all physicians on the staff or restricted to a few. The following McAuley physician's comments underscore the issue:

> Exclusivity is an issue, and it depends on who you talk to as to what sort of an issue it is. To give you an example, the radiologists have an exclusive contract with us. At the moment, that has not been an issue of concern. However, nonradiologists are beginning to do things like ultrasound, and this has created some tension between the urologists and the institution because we're honoring the exclusive arrangement with the radiologists. . . . We've also had a question involving nephrology services, but the medical staff

executive committee has looked at that and decided that the exclusive arrangement was the appropriate way to go. So while it percolates to the surface every once in a while, the executive committee has usually resolved it in favor of the arrangement. The institution has a general policy that they're not going to enter into exclusive arrangements unless the medical staff thinks it's appropriate.

Scripps Memorial Hospital

Scripps has had variable experience with its joint ventures. An early physician office building was offered as a joint venture to physicians, but the physicians believed the hospital made it very difficult for the physicians to own their own suite. The hospital is now working with XIMED (the physician organization) in developing a second physician office building on the hospital's campus. The hospital is leasing the land to a XIMED–Scripps Memorial partnership that will develop the property and manage the building. This arrangement has worked well to date. The hospital also has joint ventures in executive health and sports medicine. In all of these efforts, great care is given to avoid exclusivity and to ensure that everyone has equal access. As expressed by one Scripps physician:

> Great care is taken to see that there's equal physician access to the joint venture. . . . We have a little problem with our Whittier Institute of Diabetes and Endocrinology Research Center. We also have an enormous problem with the eye institute in that we really haven't been able to get the research going that it was funded for because of the opposition of ophthalmologists to a guy who's doing retina research. They claim it's going to be unfair competition for those doing retinal ophthalmology, and we're struggling with that issue.

Scripps has developed the following six guidelines for considering joint venture initiatives.

1. It must be mutually advantageous to both the hospital and physicians. Their must be either strategic or technical advantages.
2. The opportunity must be thoroughly analyzed with a detailed business plan containing numerous "what if?" scenarios and a two-year break-even plan or reasons why the break-even period should be longer.
3. The venture must not compromise the hospital's 501(c)3 tax-exempt status.

4. The venture must support the private practice of medicine. The hospital board has adopted a written policy indicating that they will not purchase physician practices.

5. Each party reserves the right to take their name off of a given facility or promotion associated with a specific joint venture.

6. A joint venture must contribute to a positive relationship with physicians.

Despite these guidelines, some Scripps respondents believe that developing effective joint ventures will continue to prove challenging. As one noted:

> I think this will be more and more of a problem over the years, and the hospital's got to be prudent and joint venture when they think they can, trying not to have a negative impact on the medical staff. But you're always going to make somebody mad, and I think that's just an inevitability. They have not done anything to date which, in my opinion, really hurt anybody. They've made people mad, but they haven't hurt anybody.

Sutter Health

Sutter, like the other sites, tries to keep its joint venture and related economic initiatives outside of hospital medical staff relationship issues. It has been generally successful in a number of ventures including the development of two imaging centers, the syndication of several ambulatory surgery centers, and the planned development (with primary care physicians) of three integrated medical campuses. Discussions involving the first imaging center took two and a half years, with much of it focused on concerns regarding exclusivity. The situation was described by one Sutter physician as follows:

> Exclusivity was a major problem when we were setting it [the imaging center] up because we first set it up without the radiologists. They felt that was extremely bad form, but then the economic realities of their ability to compete led to their inclusion as general partners and nobody was excluded in terms of limited partnerships. So I don't think that really became a problem. In fact, to specifically address some of those issues, some of the subspecialty units were very worried about our group practice development. They were worried what that might mean to them economically in the future. By enabling them to be heavy investors in the joint venture, their own private income needs were met. . . . Our own group is going to proceed along the same lines as the

hospital. We're going to do what we have to do, and we're doing it with as much openness as we can and as much availability to those who wish to join us. But I don't know how that's going to fall out. You know, . . . it may lead to huge confrontations. It may not. Others may appreciate that this is really the way things need to go and fall into it, so I honestly don't know how that's going to work out.

Overall, the hospital views joint ventures as another way of involving physicians and continuing to build trusting relationships. This is apparent in the comments of the following Sutter physician:

I think the major point is the willingness of the administration to cooperate with physicians to participate in these joint ventures. The willingness to say that we're going to be equal partners and that they are not going to subjugate us. I think there is significant trust between the hospital staff, administration, and physician staff. You've got to have a proven track record that you've done things successfully. One of the successful images that Sutter has is the capability in its administration and management.

The hospital also recognizes the importance of the joint venture strategy in situations where physicians threaten to develop a new service by themselves or undertake additional ancillary services testing that removes income from the hospital, as reflected in the comments of the following physician:

Those [physicians] who are innovative are looking for other means to generate income, and right now procedures still reward you the best. And if it's a simple piece of equipment and they can do it in their office, they're going to do it. The hospital knows that, and there's really nothing the physician's going to give up unless, and here's the key, the hospital says, I'll buy that equipment for you. . . . Let's do a joint venture. . . . If there's no such joint venture, then the physician's going to do it and some groups will joint venture and some groups won't.

Tucson Medical Center

The objectives of Tucson Medical Center (TMC) joint venture activities are to

1. enhance relationships between the hospital and physicians
2. secure new sources of revenue
3. afford flexibility to do things that cannot be done in other ways

Among the primary advantages that they have experienced to date are

1. an increase in the availability of capital
2. the provision of stability in unstable times
3. the sharing of risks
4. increased commitment to making things succeed

Most of their problems have been associated with the threat to physician independence since the joint ventures require a sharing of power and control, along with ego problems involving selected individuals. They have also faced exclusivity issues in forming the physician-hospital organization—a joint venture umbrella structure arrangement between the Southern Arizona Independent Physicians (SAIP) and the Medical Center. Operating under the principle of "right of first refusal," all joint venture proposals are taken to the PHO for review and a decision. But the physicians who are not a part of SAIP feel excluded. These concerns are expressed in the following comments of a TMC physician:

> I think that exclusivity is definitely a problem, particularly with the formation of the Southern Arizona Independent Physicians group. I think there are going to be some negatives to that in that some people are going to feel left out. The hospital and the SAIP are probably happy to leave them out, but there's going to be others who are going to be in the middle who may feel excluded. This is due to the development of this HMO thing, where you can't bring everybody in at once. So some people are going to be temporarily excluded, and this may create a problem unless we move along a little quicker.

Yet, by and large, most participants are optimistic that the problems can be handled. As one noted:

> I think exclusivity's been successfully dealt with. The big thing is the joining of the hospital and SAIP to form the PHO and then the PHO owning the Northwest Community Center. . . . That kind of thing is going to be an income producer for physicians as years go on. It might not be dollars this week, but it will be a worthwhile effort.

In addition to the primary care clinic, TMC has a joint venture sports medicine clinic, an imaging center, and a retirement center. They believe their future success will depend on the continued trust and credibility of the parties involved and focusing on what they do best. As expressed by one participant, "When dollars are involved, theory ends."

Crouse-Irving Memorial Hospital

Crouse-Irving Memorial has formed a task force to consider joint ventures. Their main experience to date has been with the development of a primary care clinic on the north edge of Syracuse. A number of physicians felt the hospital's intentions were not clearly communicated to the staff. As noted by one:

> Now I'm one of the beneficiaries of it [the primary care clinic], so I don't have much of a bitch about it, but I know that some of my colleagues do. A lot of them feel like things were already done, that things were already shaped up before it was even brought up. They feel that things were done in smoke-filled rooms. That creates this whole image of people not having any control and not being consulted, which reinforces other concerns people have.

Crouse-Irving Memorial has also withdrawn from a joint venture involving a mammography clinic because they felt their involvement was not needed. For the future they want to explore the possibility of a joint venture multispecialty group practice as a way of dealing better with anticipated growth in managed care. Most of those interviewed, however, felt they were at least five years away from making this a reality.

Leonard Morse Hospital

Leonard Morse has two joint ventures: one involving a walk-in center and the other a home oxygen company. The walk-in center is a joint venture between the hospital, a physician group, and a private entity. The home oxygen company involves three hospital pulmonologists as providers, with additional investment from the Allied Enterprises and Medical Services (AEMS) physician organization as a whole. It has already succeeded in attracting an additional physician from a competing hospital. Their successful experiences have benefited from an earlier negative experience in which exclusivity concerns were an issue. As related by one physician:

> The first time we tried a joint venture, it did not work because the hospital took a unilateral approach and the physicians they recruited to serve on the joint venture committee did not represent the staff. So it fell through and now is being rewired. The question is, how can we do a joint venture together? It came out of the joint conference at the last trustee meeting. My advice to the hospital is to do it with the AEMS Corporation [the physician organization].

This is the mechanism and not every physician has to participate in every joint venture. . . . Some physicians are really reluctant to put their money in things. I think a good sound proposal should go though, especially with the younger generation.

The PHO is currently being used primarily for HMO contracting.

A general reluctance of some Leonard Morse physicians to enter into business relationships with the hospital is expressed by one member:

Most doctors are not businessmen by heart. And if you put us into a room with administrators—before the dust settles my pocket is going to be empty and yours are going to be filled.

Providence Medical Center

With the exception of a network of hospital-sponsored satellite primary care group practices started in the late 1970s, Providence has limited joint venture involvement. In part this may be due to the absence of an IPA or PHO structure for considering such activity. The primary care centers, however, have developed into successful practices over time and are now an important source of specialist referrals and hospital admissions. Respondents indicated that any future joint venture initiatives would be open to all and that the hospital is very sensitive to exclusivity concerns.

West Allis Memorial

West Allis also has limited joint venture activity. They have provided financial incentives to recruit primary care physicians to a satellite primary care clinic (similar to Crouse-Irving Memorial). The hospital consulted with the appropriate physicians in advance and offered them the opportunity to expand their practices into the area before going ahead with outside physicians. As a result, no one felt left out.

Lexington Medical Center

Lexington's opportunities for joint venture involvement are legally restricted by their status as a county district hospital. They do have a lease-back arrangement with a group of cardiologists regarding the operation of an Echo machine. To the extent they are able to do joint ventures in the future, they want to target loyal physicians as primary candidates, and only then if it is necessary to have both parties involved.

North Monroe Hospital

North Monroe has no joint ventures at present. They discussed the possibility of a joint MRI but declined because it might be perceived by physicians as favoring one group over another. This occurred at a time in which the hospital was still trying to woo physicians away from a major competing hospital. The situation was described by a North Monroe executive as follows:

> The reason for not doing it is the fear we've had in terms of the other hospital. We're trying to build strong physician relationships with everyone. If we wanted investor groups of physicians, it would become more of a "we versus they" situation and we decided not to do that. The physicians basically helped me to decide that. They felt that if they became investors in this project, it might effect their referrals and, in fact, not be beneficial to the hospital.

To the extent that managed care competition grows in the area, the existence of the on-campus Northern Louisiana Clinic offers a nucleus for hospital-physician joint venture activity. The hospital realizes that it would have to be carefully structured in order to avoid exclusivity concerns with the rest of the staff.

SOME COMMON OBSERVATIONS

A number of commonalities exist in the above experiences. These include the major reasons for undertaking joint venture activities; the importance of avoiding exclusivity and of having multiple investors; the difficulty involved in developing successful joint ventures when dealing with competing groups of physicians; the importance of developing explicit criteria for reviewing initiatives including, in particular, the development of a detailed business plan; and the advantage of using a physician-hospital organization or related organizational mechanism for processing joint venture proposals.

Among the most frequently mentioned reasons for undertaking joint venture activities were

1. to increase patient referrals and revenue sources
2. to extend the continuum of care and facilitate moving patients out of the hospital into less costly and more appropriate treatment settings
3. to bond physicians closer to the hospital and build stronger, more trusting relationships

4. to pursue initiatives consistent with the strategic objectives of both hospitals and physicians

5. to present physicians with alternatives to developing activities on their own that might be competitive with the hospital

These objectives were not limited to the ten study sites. For example, a useful statement of joint venture policy is expressed by Presbyterian Healthcare Services (PHS) Albuquerque, New Mexico, in Exhibit 12.1.

Avoiding exclusivity is paramount. As underscored by one McAuley executive, "It's a huge mistake to exclude people." Given developing concerns over conflict of interest in regard to patient referrals to facilities where physicians have an economic interest, most sites found it important to dilute physician investment by attracting additional outside investors. While recognizing the conflict-of-interest issue, all sites planned to continue to explore joint venture opportunities and saw them as an important component of building the relationship. There was also some suggestion that joint venture arrangements might be associated with less Medicare fraud and abuse because of the generally higher quality people, higher accountability standards, and closer oversight associated with most joint venture activity.

The need for a common set of criteria, including a detailed business plan, was an evolving process in most sites. This was often facilitated by

Exhibit 12.1   Statement of Joint Venture Policy of Presbyterian Healthcare Services, Albuquerque, New Mexico

---

PHS/Physician Relationships: Policy Statement

PHS will develop innovative mechanisms which closely integrate PHS and physicians, promote mutual loyalty and interdependence, and facilitate mutual competitive positioning.

Background

Historically, relationships between PHS and its physicians have been constructive. The organized medical staff has fulfilled its delegated responsibilities, while individual physicians have generally been the primary determinants of their practice decisions and economics. The hospital has provided facilities and personnel to serve physicians and their patients. Conflicts which have arisen have usually been appropriately addressed because of overriding pateint care motivations and the good will of the involved parties who have recognized their informal interdependence.

Today the historical relationship of PHS and its physicians is threatened and rapidly changing. Size, complexity and the pace of change challenge historical values and relationships, but most of all the economics of healthcare place increased

---

Continued

Exhibit 12.1 Continued

pressure on all parties. The healthcare financial pie is being contained in its dollar growth by government, business and consumers while an increasing number of providers (physicians, hospitals and alternative delivery setting providers) compete for the available patients and dollars. As a result, mechanisms that link physicians and hospitals and financing in order to deliver specified care to a group of patients are rapidly emerging phenomena.

In anticipation of the impact of the increasingly competitive environment on the traditional physician/hospital relationship, the physician relationships task force in 1982 adopted several recommendations regarding same as part of the strategic planning process. Those principles, such as shared risks and profits, integrated business operations to achieve competitive advantages, and shared responsibility for market development, were more prudent responses to the new competitive environment than was the unrecognized interdependence of the past. Among the guidelines specified regarding the development of economic relationships between SCHS and its phsyicians were:

- Innovative hospital-physician relationship to achieve market and financial objectives may be developed separately from existing medical staff arrangements.
- Innovative relationships may be tailored to meet the particular needs of individual physicians or physician groups and need not be uniform or appropriate to all staff members.
- Joint ventures with shared risk/reward are encouraged. Arrangements to be considered may include: shared ownership of healthcare resources (i.e., professional office buildings, surgi-centers, urgent care centers, etc.) and/or shared risk/reward for the operation of healthcare services (i.e., contract hospital or ambulatory care, alcohol rehabilitation, etc.).
- The common objective of all new arrangements should be the provision of quality care and the maintenance or enhancement of the competitive and financial positions of SCHS hospitals and physicians.

The transition state—from principles to their actual implementation—has been a valuable experience as the particular details, working relationships and ramifications of various ventures have played out. Among the experiences SCHS/PHS have had in physician-hospital arrangements are urgent care centers, Cooperative Health Care (the preferred provider organization) and the Magnetic Resonance Imaging (MRI) project. Although each has been unique, their development has, for the most part, incorporated the physician relationships task force's principles and recommendations. There also are projects originally cited by the task force (e.g., surgi-center joint ventures) that have not been aggressively pursued for a number of reasons.

Recognizing the continued need to respond appropriately to patient care needs and market opportunities, SCHS/PHS anticipates and welcomes venture opportunities allowing SCHS to invest resources to support its physicians. All such potential ventures will be critically examined from the perspective of the physician relationships task force recommendations; they also must be found to further the overall PHS mission.

Continued

Exhibit 12.1   Continued

PHS Mission

Presbyterian Healthcare Services is a network of organizations joined together to provide patient centered, high quality, cost-effective hospital and health-related services to residents of the Greater Albuquerque area and to serve as the referral center for New Mexico and the surrounding region.

In order to achieve the PHS mission and implement the physician relationships policy, PHS shall:

- Take initiative to determine PHS' role in the healthcare market including organization and investment in alternative delivery systems based on the considered judgment of the board of trustees;
- Enter joint ventures, economic investments and other mutually beneficial arrangements with selected PHS physicians who demonstrate commitment to PHS; and
- Select as partners in specific ventures PHS physicians who demonstrate interest in a stronger cooperative relationship and who meet general criteria, to include credentialling, good patient care, cost-effective practice, initiative and demonstrated commitment to PHS.

Membership on the PHS medical staff is a separate and distinct privilege from participation in the various arrangements referred to above.

Southwest Community Health Services and Presbyterian Healthcare Services will take the initiative to determine the role PHS hospitals will play in the healthcare system and will allocate where appropriate resources to support this policy.

Reprinted with the permission of Presbyterian Healthcare Services.

the development of the physician-hospital organization as the organizational forum for considering such activities. This organization also helped in sorting out the issues between two or more physician groups who were in conflict with each other. The most frequent conflicts appeared to involve cardiology and orthopedic groups. The PHO would often act as an intermediary in helping to resolve such conflict and facilitate both groups seeing the benefits of joint collaboration.

TORRANCE MEMORIAL: A MINICASE

Many of the study's observations are illustrated in a novel way by the business relationship developed between Torrance Memorial Hospital, Torrance, California, and its physicians. Their experience as reported in *Healthcare Organization Report* (Brice 1989) is described below.*

---

*The Torrance Memorial Hospital minicase on pages 183–95 is reprinted with permission from *Healthcare Organization Report*, Volume 2 (January 1989), published by COR Research, Inc., Santa Barbara, CA.

Torrance Memorial Hospital, through the formation of Health Access Systems (HAS) in 1984, sold the rights to the revenue stream of most of its outpatient services to its medical staff.

The result has been a seven-point increase in the hospital's market share and a significant return on investment for the hospital-physician joint venture. HAS has allowed the hospital to collect more than $8 million in cash it would otherwise not have had for business development activities.

The architects of the scheme they call the Torrance Model are George Graham, chief executive officer of Torrance Memorial Hospital, his chief financial officer, Ray Rahn, and Douglas Mancino, partner in the law firm of McDermott Will & Emery.

Health Access Systems adds up to more than the sum of its parts. While typical joint ventures are limited to small, targeted physician groups, HAS bonds most of Torrance Memorial's physicians to the hospital through a master partnership shared equally by Torrance Memorial and its 140 physician partners.

HAS encourages referrals through eight secondary joint ventures. Ownership is shared with subgroups of practitioners who are most likely to refer patients to the services.

But the Torrance Model's most revolutionary feature is the purchase of 20-year rights to revenue streams generated by outpatient services. Thus, while typical joint ventures make major equipment purchases that duplicate assets already available in the hospital, HAS makes use of those existing assets.

Consequently, HAS's business development costs were lower, and its prospects for financial success were higher than conventional venturing arrangements. It was expected to pull in about $2.6 million on revenue of $12 million in 1988, according to Rahn. The return on investment on its secondary joint ventures in 1987 ranged between 20 percent and a phenomenal 106 percent.

Financial Pressures

Like most novel ideas, this innovation was mothered by necessity. The 330-bed Torrance Memorial Hospital was on about equal footing with Little Company of Mary, a 268-bed Catholic hospital, and the 203-bed South Bay Hospital, a district facility that had recently been purchased by American Medical International, Inc., a for-profit chain. South Bay had a 20 percent share of both inpatient and outpatient services. Torrance and Little Company each had about a 40 percent market share.

Some 700 physicians served this community of 400,000 people, located 30 miles southwest of Los Angeles. Most practitioners used all three hospitals. Yet, according to Graham, fewer than 200 physicians accounted for 80 percent of Torrance Memorial's admissions. Although Medicare DRGs were just being implemented, it was already clear to Graham that outpatient services were essential to his hospital's financial growth.

Yet, Torrance's business-minded physician community was also attuned to opportunities in outpatient care. A physician-owned surgery center was already in business across the street. Many other ventures were in the planning, according to Rahn.

"We had some entrepreneurial doctors here who thought the hospital had no place in life other than housing intensive care," he said. "All other services could be handled on an outpatient basis, and those services could be owned by the physicians themselves."

It didn't require much thought, according to Rahn, to realize that Torrance Memorial couldn't survive if critical care became its primary source of income. "It was apparent that these proposed joint ventures would siphon off our highest-margin business," Rahn stressed.

Broadly Based Response

Torrance Memorial's response to these conditions was hashed out around a conference table during long evening meetings between Graham, Rahn, and Mancino. Market share was the central issue during these discussions: how to hold on to patient volume threatened by the new physician-sponsored services being planned, while gaining an upper hand on Torrance Memorial's traditional competition.

It became clear the hospital needed a broadly based plan that would engage as many physicians as possible. And it needed to move quickly to get Torrance Memorial's own program implemented before the physicians committed their money and loyalty to the host of outside alternatives being planned.

"The hospital had to be proactive," Mancino said. "The opportunity to take a stand would have, otherwise, passed the hospital by entirely."

A venture capital corporation that purchased the rights to the revenue stream from Torrance Memorial's existing outpatient services met both these needs. HAS made a one-time payment for the rights to profits and losses generated by specific outpatient services during the next 20 years. The hospital retained title to the assets and continued to control all aspects of departmental management. HAS would pay Torrance Memorial direct and indirect costs for the departments through user fees.

Dangerous Legal Waters

Selling the rights to the profits and losses to specific product lines within a hospital was an entirely new idea, according to Graham, one which treads dangerous legal waters, especially considering Torrance Memorial's nonprofit status.

"Maintaining nonprofit status became the acid test on whether this project would fly," Graham stressed. Torrance Memorial's 501(c)(3) designation exempted the hospital from state and federal corporate income taxes and local property taxes, and allowed for tax-exempt financing. The value of these privileges outweighed any gains Torrance Memorial could make from the proposed venture, Graham said.

The nonprofit question was so compelling and the proposed contract was so complex that Torrance Memorial needed an unprecedented letter ruling from the Internal Revenue Service (IRS) before proceeding with the plan.

Two issues were critical for IRS approval, according to Mancino. One concerned inurement: whether the nonprofit's assets would financially enrich the proposed for-profit enterprise. The other related to whether the proposal was consistent with Memorial's nonprofit mission of community service.

The inurement issue was dealt with by assuring the IRS that Health Access would pay the fair market value for the revenue streams. Valuation Counselers, Inc., Los Angeles, calculated $1.3 million to be the fair market value for the revenue streams for outpatient surgery, cardiac nuclear medicine, diagnostic services, and outpatient ophthalmic services, the four outpatient services that would originally comprise the HAS product line.

Rahn answered the community service question by showing how additional volume anticipated from the sale would help Torrance Memorial control the price of healthcare. "Because we are largely a fixed-cost institution, we could keep our charges down by increasing volume through these joint-ventured services," Rahn said.

Mancino recalled that Rahn drew an analogy between a pie and the hospital to illustrate his point. The hospital could own 100 percent of a 6-inch diameter pie, or it could own 96 percent of a 7-inch pie. "As volume increased, its incremental fixed costs could be spread among more admissions," Mancino said. "This meant charges could either be controlled or decline."

Four months passed before the IRS approved the initial plan, according to Mancino. A second letter ruling was needed when HAS was expanded to other outpatient services. That approval took five weeks.

Physicians Buy In

Health Access Systems was incorporated as a general business corporation and C-corporation for tax purposes in November 1984. All physicians on the hospital's medical staff were given an opportunity to buy stock in the new company. Torrance Memorial matched their investment dollar-for-dollar to gain a 50 percent interest in the new corporation. Its investment assured the hospital control of three of the six seats on HAS's governing board of directors.

The sale of HAS stock generated more equity and physician participation than was expected, according to Graham. The California Department of Corporations had authorized the sale of $1.4 million in stock to be matched by the hospital's contribution. The physicians actually contributed $1.74 million. Individuals could invest no less than $7,500 and no more than $30,000. The offering was limited to Torrance Memorial's medical staff.

The sale assured HAS the broad physician involvement its founders sought for the organization. "We wanted a democratic mechanism to allow physicians who didn't have a direct professional interest in the services sold to the venture to also get involved," Mancino noted. "We were conscious of the political ramifications of dealing with physicians who were left out."

Physicians excluded from participating in HAS could easily have defected to similar offerings posed by Torrance Memorial's competition. In fact, Little Company of Mary formed a hospital-physician joint venture for Del Amo Diagnostic Center, a $15 million, freestanding multiservice facility, at about the same time.

"We intended to make the physicians take sides," Mancino said.

Dr. Marshall Davis, a radiation oncologist with Del Amo Diagnostic Center, lends evidence that Torrance Memorial's strategy worked. "Right now, doctors tied to the Torrance Memorial joint ventures use that facility to the exclusion of us," he said. Davis also noted that Torrance Memorial aggressively recruited younger physicians a couple of years ago. Those physicians now have built their practices and are contributing volume to that hospital. That's something that Little Company didn't do, he acknowledged.

Secondary Joint Ventures

Following Torrance Memorial's initial stock sale, another $1 million was raised in August 1985 by forming separate subsidiary joint ventures around each of the four product lines comprising the investment with

Torrance Memorial. Though these investment opportunities were limited to HAS's stockholders, the partners in these cases were drawn from medical specialties most likely to "enhance" referrals to the services, according to Graham.

Four additional services from the hospital and associated joint ventures were added later, producing another $1.56 million in equity for HAS. Outpatient diagnostic services were reorganized under HAS in 1985. Two limited partnerships were formed in mid-1987, for outpatient cardiology and noninvasive cardiac rehabilitation, and for the hospital's catheterization lab. HAS acquired an outpatient magnetic resonance imaging (MRI) center in July 1987 and converted the business to a limited partnership in January 1988. HAS holds a 50 percent interest in each venture, while physician limited partners share the remaining 50 percent.

Radiation therapy and physical therapy are currently the only major outpatient services not syndicated through HAS, according to planning director Sally Eberhard. She said the hospital retained those services because of their limited potential for profit and physician referral. But their status will again be reviewed in 1989.

No Change in Management

The responsibility for making this new system work is shared between the hospital's management, which retained control over all aspects of outpatient services, and the physician investors, whose referrals are essential to the services' growth. Equipment, personnel, labor relations, managed care contracting, productivity management, and quality assurance all remained under the hospital's control, according to Graham.

"My fellow CEOs often ask me who manages this mess?" Graham said. "Well, it really isn't a mess. It's really clean. Ostensibly, there is no change in management."

It is impossible for patients to ascertain that their physicians have an economic interest in some services housed within the hospital. The hospital has avoided extreme conflict-of-interest problems by limiting the joint ventures to outpatient services. That distinction means that patients admitted to the hospital will not cross the invisible line between hospital-owned services and services supported by physician investments during their stays.

Prescriptions to outpatient services carry a printed notice informing the patient that the referring physician owns part of the service being prescribed. The patient is told that another similar service is available, if he or she wishes.

HAS also remains on the legal side of Medicare's stringent fraud and abuse law by basing physician dividends solely on the joint ventures' financial performance, according to HAS board chairman Dr. Warren Hoffman. The diverse composition of HAS's physician ownership further strengthens its position with respect to the law.

Because HAS paid fair market value of the revenue streams, their value to the master joint venture depended upon additional volume generated through physician referral, according to Graham. "The only benefit they (the physician partners) may gain through ownership can come by growing the business," he noted.

How do physicians in the area view Torrance Memorial's arrangements? Dr. Davis, who is associated with Little Company of Mary, noted that "there are physicians in Torrance who don't think joint ventures are a good idea. There are even physicians in joint ventures who don't want to feel the pressure to use the facility," he said. "Some doctors are involved in joint ventures just because they think it's a good investment."

But Dr. Davis believes that most physicians in Torrance "go where the care is best. Here, as elsewhere," he said, "physicians place the interests of their patients first, before other considerations." To attract so much business, the facilities at Torrance Memorial have to be first rate.

Accounting Complications

While medical care is dispensed smoothly, the administration of the hospital and joint ventures from an accounting standpoint is exceedingly complex [Figure 12.1]. Outpatient service technicians are hospital employees, paid through Torrance Memorial's payroll system. However, most of the services they provide are for Health Access. The formula for calculating Health Access's equitable share of their expense is spelled out in the user agreement between HAS and Torrance Memorial. The accounting system must isolate those costs on an item-by-item basis.

Graham, Rahn, and other hospital administrators also split their time between HAS and Torrance Memorial. Consequently, the allocation of indirect costs they generate is difficult.

"We decided from Day 1 to give HAS its own accounting department," Rahn said. "We started with one accountant. He now has a four-person staff."

Mutual trust is essential to make such a complex business relationship work, according to Rahn. While HAS owns the revenue, the authority to negotiate managed care contracts, set prices, and determine

Figure 12.1 Organizational Structure for Torrance Health Association

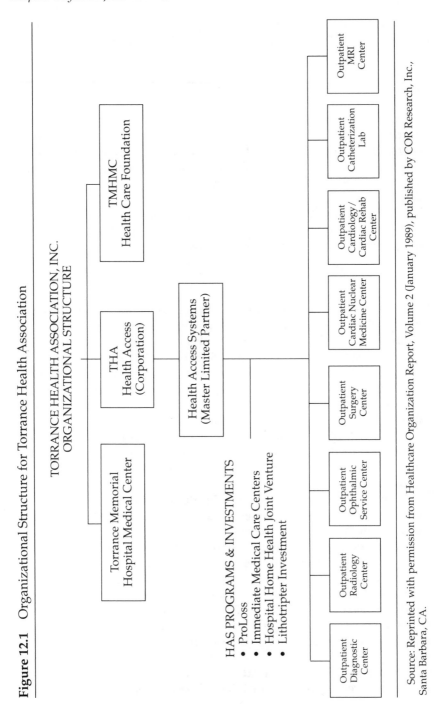

TORRANCE HEALTH ASSOCIATION, INC.
ORGANIZATIONAL STRUCTURE

Torrance Memorial Hospital Medical Center

THA Health Access (Corporation)

TMHMC Health Care Foundation

Health Access Systems (Master Limited Partner)

HAS PROGRAMS & INVESTMENTS
- ProLoss
- Immediate Medical Care Centers
- Hospital Home Health Joint Venture
- Lithotripter Investment

Outpatient Diagnostic Center

Outpatient Radiology Center

Outpatient Ophthalmic Service Center

Outpatient Surgery Center

Outpatient Cardiac Nuclear Medicine Center

Outpatient Cardiology/ Cardiac Rehab Center

Outpatient Catheterization Lab

Outpatient MRI Center

Source: Reprinted with permission from Healthcare Organization Report, Volume 2 (January 1989), published by COR Research, Inc., Santa Barbara, CA.

labor rates rests with the hospital. Although the physicians own half of Health Access, Graham wields considerable authority over business ventures HAS pursues."

Individual physicians wouldn't have invested up to $30,000 in this enterprise if they didn't have confidence that management would be able to represent their interests," Rahn said.

Graham believes his administration passed a major test of physician trust in 1987 when it recommended that HAS drop its status as a general corporation in favor of a master limited partnership. The 1986 Tax Reform Act, which would have subjected physician income from HAS to double taxation, led to the recommendation, according to Mancino.

"Only one physician voted against the motion," Graham noted, "so they were nearly unanimous in supporting the hospital when we said that this change was in their interest."

Conflict Over MRI

Health Access's central mission is to maximize its return on investment for physicians, according to Graham, while Torrance Memorial's mission is to be a full-service hospital serving the local community. This difference leads to conflicts, especially when selecting projects the hospital and joint ventures will pursue.

"The hospital can be much more gregarious in going after new technology," Graham said, "where Health Access is more cold and calculated."

That was initially the case with magnetic resonance imaging. The hospital dropped plans to buy into this expensive new technology about three years ago because HAS physician stockholders opposed it on financial grounds.

The hospital and physicians flip-flopped positions in 1988. This time the physicians championed MRI while Graham and Rahn argued the acquisition would be a loser.

"But the physicians felt the equipment was needed and were willing to risk money to get it," Dr. Hoffman said.

"This was one case where the physicians' judgment was better than ours," Graham admitted. "We didn't realize so many applications for MRI would become available. The returns have exceeded expectations."

Graham said the hospital leases the top-of-the-line General Electric imager. HAS reimburses Torrance Memorial for its share of machine use.

Some physicians objected to Graham's decision to purchase an urgent-care center for HAS in 1986. "One member of the medical staff threatened to burn it down, because he saw it as direct competition to his own practice," he remembered. "Well, we bought it anyway, which means this physician invested in it and now benefits from its performance."

HAS credited the center with 300 new patient referrals to physicians affiliated with HAS in 1987. On the strength of its performance, a second similar facility at Rancho Palos Verdes was organized in mid-1988.

Informal Communications

HAS's physician investors almost exclusively use informal channels to affect decision-making. "We encourage physicians to bring their ideas to our attention," Graham said. He noted that HAS invested heavily into mammography at the physicians' urging. Its Breast Diagnosis Center, which has just been equipped with its third mammographer, is one of HAS's most successful enterprises.

Although the physicians' ownership of such equipment is limited to the revenue it produces, they have a "feeling of ownership" in these facilities, according to Mark Costa, Torrance Memorial 's vice president of administration. "That's the biggest change I've seen since Health Access was started," he said.

This feeling of ownership, Costa notes, means physicians are more likely to speak up when they see how services can be improved. For example, evening hours were established for the Breast Diagnosis Center after management learned through referring physicians that daytime appointments were inconvenient for working patients.

The physicians' suggestions are also more realistic than before Health Access was formed, according to Costa. "HAS has opened the physicians' ears to what it takes to profitably run these departments," he said. "The quality demands of physicians who don't have a financial stake in these services can be never-ending."

Good Performance

Physician confidence in HAS has been encouraged by its performance. Torrance Memorial's market share rose seven points during Health Access's first three years, according to Rahn. Through the first nine months of 1988, patient days increased 11 percent over the same period in 1987. Patient days at Little Company of Mary and South Bay Hospital declined 4.4 percent and 2.6 percent respectively. HAS's performance and Torrance Memorial's success in managed care contracting are both credited for those gains.

In 1984, the combined revenues of the four services initially sold to HAS totaled $2.9 million. Pre-tax net earnings were $183,000, according to Graham. Revenues rose to $4.5 million with pre-tax earnings of $989,000 in the next year.

In addition to its share of profits, the hospital recovered $1 million in fees charged to the venture. "In essence, the hospital enjoyed the full financial benefit experienced prior to the divestitures," Graham noted.

Units of the master limited partnership which sold for $10 in 1984 have a current book value of $15.60, according to Rahn. Three dividends totaling $3.30 per unit have been paid in addition to dividend distributions from secondary joint ventures.

New Investments

Most of HAS's profits, however, have been poured back into the business. "The whole purpose of divesting the revenue streams from the hospital was to develop a core business that would engender close cooperation between physicians and the hospital," Graham said. "It was not intended to be an end in itself, but a starting point to pursue new services and acquire existing ones."

The urgent-care centers and mammography equipment were two of those new investments. ProLoss, a weight reduction program, and Home Health Ventures, Inc. were others. HAS also invested in a lithotripter installed at Memorial Hospital of Long Beach. "We didn't have to spend $2 million to gain access to this technology," Dr. Hoffman noted, "but we were able to gain a share of this equipment (which disintegrates kidney stones with high-energy shock waves) with the proviso that our urologists could use it."

Torrance Memorial has also made improvements in services shared with HAS. A new colorflow dopler unit and computerized EKG were acquired for the newly remodeled outpatient cardiology department. The radiology department was renovated. Plans are underway to break ground for a new cardiac catheterization lab before the end of 1988.

Torrance Memorial spent about $2.5 million for new equipment in 1988. Graham estimates the hospital will invest another $25 million for all projects currently being readied for construction.

HAS helps the hospital gain a return on investment from these facilities in two ways, according to Costa. It first adds volume through outpatient services. And, because its equipment is located at the hospital, HAS encourages the physicians to increase their utilization of inpatient services. The equipment's fixed costs are distributed over more units of care; consequently the profit margins are larger.

Graham believes he's in a far stronger position to react to changing market conditions than before HAS was formed. In his opinion, HAS is a much more flexible, leaner organization than the hospital. Graham is one of only six people to sit on the HAS board. The hospital's own board of trustees has 25 members.

"Health Access has fewer constituencies to satisfy." Graham said. "It is oriented toward taking more risks."

In 1989, Graham intends to backtrack a bit to accommodate one of Health Access's inherent limitations. The supply of HAS shares has not kept up with the number of new doctors who have joined the hospital since the first sale of stock, despite the fact that physicians are obligated to sell their interests when they drop their medical privileges with Torrance Memorial, retire, or die. HAS's growth solves that problem at least for now. It will permit a secondary stock offering to the hospital's new blood, according to Graham, without diluting the value of the original investments.

Graham also faces the problem of saturating the local market. Although HAS continues to examine additional acquisitions and start-up opportunities, Graham admits, "Our plate is quite full right now."

Replicating the Model

So, what's in store for the future of this synthesis of venture capitalism and health care joint venturing? "We're looking for opportunities to network," said Dr. Hoffman. "We're getting the word out on what we've accomplished here to create consulting opportunities to replicate this model elsewhere."

HAS's mating instincts first took it to Washington State where it helped Seattle's Northwest Hospital establish Pacific Consolidated Corporation. In addition to a consulting contract, Health Access has a 5 percent equity interest in its first offspring. Pacific Consolidated made its first securities offering in 1987.

Northwest Hospital is certainly not the only facility to be in the competitive position Torrance Memorial faced in 1984. Market share is an issue wherever there's a cross-town hospital. This new business framework for medical care may be a model to be replicated, especially for nonprofit hospitals cut off from other means of capital formation.

PROS AND CONS OF THE TORRANCE MODEL

In their book, *Joint Ventures Between Hospitals and Physicians,* Douglas Mancino and co-author Linda A. Burns [1986] draw distinctions between typical joint ventures and the kind of venture capital company that the Torrance Model proposes.

They note that most joint ventures are designed to raise funds for direct participation in a single project. The venture capital company, however, has as its primary purpose the raising of funds for investment in several projects of interest to both hospitals and physicians. In fact, venture capital projects or businesses frequently may be defined only in general terms at the time the funds are raised.Venture capital companies differ from Medical Staff Hospital Joint Ventures (MeSH), first proposed by Paul Ellwood of InterStudy in Minneapolis. Unlike the MeSH, the venture capital company is intended to focus on new business development, rather than on alternative delivery system and insurance types of contractual arrangements.

Advantages of the Torrance Model

1. For hospitals, it is an uncomplicated way to get participation from all its medical staff in a true, economic risk-sharing joint venture.

2. For the physicians, it is an uncomplicated way of pooling substantial resources to engage in various business development opportunities.

3. It is a means of spreading financial risk among a large number of investors and a broad range of investments. The downside risk of losing money on one project may be offset by the upside potential for profit on others.

4. It creates opportunities for two-tiered investment. The venture capital company is the first tier. On the second tier are secondary joint ventures tailored to appeal to narrower segments of the medical staff. These ventures are created either through stock sales in corporate subsidiaries or interests in partnerships in which the venture capital company is the general partner.

Disadvantages

1. The venture capital company will likely be unable to distance itself from hospital-medical staff conflicts and problems enough to make it truly independent.

2. There may be great difficulty in approaching business development objectively. Lack of objectivity is likely to arise both in the selection of business development opportunities and in dealing with operational problems.

3. The types of business undertaken by the venture capital company may not support the development of marketing, finance, and other support functions.

4. Shareholders of the venture capital company will be the true owners of the corporation and its underlying assets. The board will need to be more responsive to the needs of the shareholders and, as a consequence, will be more subject to pressure from individual shareholders.

JOINT VENTURE BEST PRACTICES

1. It is important that both the hospital and physicians be at financial risk. Financial accountability means that the activity will receive serious and ongoing attention from both parties. Research on joint ventures in other industries confirms that risk sharing is a key factor influencing success (Chakravarthy and Zajac 1984; Demski 1976; Rumelt 1987).

2. The joint ventures should provide strategic fit with both the hospital's and physicians' plans. Ideally, it should be an outgrowth of the strategic planning process involving both physicians and the hospital.

3. There should be explicit review criteria that include the development of a detailed business plan with a realistic forecast of revenues and expenses and contingency plans for "pulling the plug" if performance does not meet expectations.

4. Exclusivity should be avoided at all costs. Opportunities should be made available to all physicians for investment. In addition, it is often important to attract outside investors both for purposes of limiting conflict of interest as well as for acquiring additional capital.

5. The joint venture should be managed as a professional business relationship.

Successful joint venture relationships require executives and physicians who can work with each other as mature business partners. To illustrate this point, it is interesting to note one executive's comments regarding the career of Ray Brown, a noted hospital executive: "He appeared to deal with the medical staff as a business peer, giving respect to their skills and getting theirs for his."

REFERENCES

Brice, J. 1989. "In a Ground-Breaking Joint Venture, Torrance Memorial Sells 20 Year Revenue Streams from Outpatient Services to Physicians," *Healthcare Organization Report* 2(1):1–8.

Burns, L. A. and D. Mancino. 1986. *Joint Ventures between Hospitals and Physicians: A Competitive Strategy for the Healthcare Marketplace*. Homewood, Il: Dow Jones–Irwin.

Chakravarthy, B., and E. J. Zajac. 1984. "Tailoring Incentive Systems to a Strategic Context," *Planning Review* 12:30–35.

Coopers and Lybrand. 1988. "The Hospital-Physician Partnership: Options for Improving Relations," *Medical Staff Relations*, pp. 131–39.

Demski, J. 1976. "Uncertainty and Evaluation Based on Controllable Performance," *Journal of Accounting Research* 10:230–45.

Rumelt, R. P. 1987. "Theory, Strategy, and Entrepreneurship," in D. J. Teece (Ed.), *The Competitive Challenge: Strategies for Industrial Innovation and Renewal*. Cambridge, MA: Ballinger, 137–58.

CHAPTER 13

Cost Containment

Somewhat surprisingly, cost containment was not reported as a major issue by most study sites. Nor was it frequently mentioned as a criterion used to judge the effectiveness of the hospital-physician relationship. Few respondents reported inappropriate or extensive pressure to discharge patients or change their admission patterns. The hospital-physician questionnaire data indicated a high degree of satisfaction with admission and discharge policies across the ten sites, with a mean rating of 4.0 and a range from 3.3 to 4.8. Most sites recognized the obvious and continued need to contain costs and, with few exceptions, had involved physicians early and continuously in the efforts to do so (Eisenberg 1986). Most sites, however, had gone beyond cost-containment activities to actively work with their physicians to enhance revenues (as discussed in the previous three chapters). The basic cost-containment approaches and practices of each site are briefly highlighted below along with some sites' approaches to malpractice insurance coverage.

TEN SITES' EXPERIENCES

Crouse-Irving Memorial Hospital

With its teaching programs, Crouse-Irving Memorial is one of the higher-cost Syracuse area hospitals operating in the highly regulated New York State environment. A resource management committee involving physicians is used to review new programs and consider possible cuts. There have been some staff cuts—primarily among security staff. The committee emphasizes that proposals must generate revenues to cover costs. There is some disagreement among the staff regarding

197

the hospital's cost-cutting approaches and their impact. One physician notes:

> It hasn't really presented any problem. . . . Our deletions of services have not been cost-containment efforts, per se. We have a nursing shortage along with a whole lot of other places. My perception is that if 50 nurses walked in the door tomorrow, we'd hire them. Cost containment has not really impacted on our medical programs.

A contrasting view is offered by a second physician:

> They [the physicians] feel that a lot of the cuts that have been made have been in areas that are vital for patient care. They see that we're getting a new lobby, and so they wonder . . . why nursing staff are being curtailed. "What is this? What we need are the people to take care of the patients." . . . I guess no one likes to see anyone lose a job, but it seems like these are vital people that we need to take care of patients. We don't understand. . . . Apparently it's different budgets that can fix our lobby, but we can't continue with the transport service people or the IV team because that's a different budget. That's hard for us to understand. I think the administration, again, needs to educate us. We had a study about three years ago where it indicated we were top heavy; we had too much staff. So they put a freeze on nursing. That's almost brought us to our knees. We have beds we can't open because we don't have nurses. We have the most beautiful ICU unit without enough nurses to staff it. . . . From the administrative view, they're doing everything they can to change that, but they had a hiring freeze. And then there's just a shortage of nurses, as you know, nationwide.

A third physician respondent noted:

> I mean the word drifts down from on high that the hospital's 3 to 12 million in the hole. And that there's going to be cost cutting. I have a big axe to grind as to which costs to cut. They're putting a $3,000 plant in the foyer when you find they're laying off critical care nurses. I'm not pleased with that. . . . I personally don't even know what they're doing to cut costs. They've talked about early retirements and this, that, and the other thing, and it may well be that at the executive committee it's been discussed at great length. But I don't know what they're doing. . . . Are they going to cut quality? I don't know. I honestly don't know what in the world they're doing to cut costs.

. . . But there's been no harm on quality. They've always been very good about that. I have to admit that's not a problem. There is a diminishing quality in terms of number of nurses, but I'm not sure that it's a financial problem in terms of if you give people raises, you will get more people. So if you don't have enough nurses, you need to get enough money so the nurses will come out of the trees.

The hospital will be devoting even more attention to staffing issues due to a recent New York State law restricting the number of hours to be worked by residents.

The hospital's relationship with its physicians has also been stained from time to time by malpractice rate concerns. Several years ago, orthopedists refused to take care of emergency room patients because of the malpractice risk. Conflict arose when administration hired another physician to provide coverage without discussing it with the orthopedists.

Leonard Morse Hospital

Leonard Morse, also operating in a highly regulated state (Massachusetts), is a relatively costly hospital in its area. While they have had no recent staff cuts, increased attention is being given to monitoring costs—especially in the area of nurse staffing. This is reflected in the following comments: "Let me tell you, at the last physician-nurse committee meeting we were talking about the nursing budget. . . . I'm telling them that they have to get their budgets under control. We're five weeks into the budget and already $55,000 over. I'm tightening up."

Leonard Morse respondents agree that more ongoing education needs to be done along with efforts to become more involved in managed care activity through their PHO. Yet at the same time, increases in malpractice rates are affecting physicians' incomes, making them more reluctant to deal with HMO discounting.

Lexington Medical Center

Lexington is one of the lower-cost hospitals in its area but, nonetheless, cut about 100 staff three years ago in closing down one patient floor. The process was handled well, with one respondent commenting: "We had worked them [the cuts] through. They didn't happen overnight. People weren't surprised." Nonetheless, some respondents noted that a "residual paranoia" still exists.

The hospital also has a utilization review process that is described by the physicians as "good and reasonable." The medical director works one-on-one with physicians on their utilization problems using comparative data. They plan to expand this effort in the future.

McAuley Health Center

Like several of the other sites, McAuley has a clinical resource committee, with heavy physician involvement, that reviews new requests. Major cuts to date have been mainly with their psychiatric hospital. This has caused some concern, as expressed by the following physician's comment:

> I have great concerns, especially since the acuity of the patient we are admitting is now higher. They're much more sick than they've ever been. . . . And then we're faced with having to cut staff and nursing. The staff-to-patient ratio has always been wonderful here, but it's going downward. It's a concern to me. They've had to hold admissions on units at times because the patients were too ill to allow anybody else that was really that ill. . . . You don't want anyone getting hurt. We've had a number of staff injured recently. We've had half of our nursing unit quit on our closed unit in the last two months because of the intensity of the patient. So I am very, very concerned. McAuley physicians also face high state malpractice insurance rates. As one approach to the problem, the Health Center has worked out a contractual relationship with obstetrician-gynecologists which enables them to obtain more reasonable coverage.

McAuley's major strategy, however, is to increase revenues by increasing volume. As one executive noted:

> Rather than cut costs and lay people off, we went the other direction. We want to control costs but with a lot of participation as appropriate and go on the upside and go after the volume. That's going against all trends.

North Monroe Hospital

In contrast to most of the sites, North Monroe has increased staff in recent years. Their main focus is on containing costs in areas that do not directly involve patient care. As one executive noted:

> I'd rather spend more money on staff and the nursing floors and do away with marketing. We really don't hard-sell advertising be-

cause I don't think there's a good return in our community. It's ineffective in our market. We make large donations to charity groups, civic groups where we've got a lot of visibility, and we've taken a lot of those dollars and put it back in to providing additional staffing or services. . . . We're also trying to be efficient. . . . If you can manage interdepartmental conflicts . . . you become more efficient.

They also involve people in setting priorities for allocation of capital from the HCA (Hospital Corporation of America) corporate office to the hospital. In response to an initial wish list, the CEO told the group:

You are the people who are requesting it, I want you to sit down with each other and come back with a list for a total of $1.3 million, and I'll give you my word that I will defend this to everybody at HCA. And what happened was that afternoon they spent four hours. They wanted to get it resolved, and they came back with a list of equipment, prioritized and why it was important, and we went with it. These people are the ones that are there on the front line.

Providence Medical Center

In response to growing financial pressures, Providence laid off approximately 30 administrative and support staff in late 1988. Some of these were associated with their primary care group practice satellite network. They are also increasing their educational efforts with physicians. As one physician commented:

We are really going to get a lot more aggressive about trying to deal with utilization management. First of all, we need to educate physicians. We're attempting to get data on practice patterns, cost, charges per patient, and so on. And, hopefully, with an educational kind of effort, we'll be able to look at why there are deviations and improve utilization of resources. . . . I also want to look at a section of the patients admitted on a regular basis and see if we can determine that the patients admitted need to be there. And, secondly, to get them out in a more timely manner. I want to do that personally for a while to get a feel for it and then turn that over to nonphysician personnel later.

Now we have a complete set of recommendations for use of prophylactic antibiotics, as an example, and a pharmacy therapeutic's committee works vigorously on the cost effectiveness of drugs. I think we need to make physicians more aware of how they're spending the money. . . . I think we have a long ways to go. We don't know the costs of the tests that the physicians are ordering. It's our responsibility to tell them, and we just haven't. Now, overall, we're probably not doing too badly because in terms of length of stay and costs, we compare favorably. We are the least-expensive hospital in our peer group. But that doesn't mean that we can't be better.

For the most part, this effort is supported by physicians, and they have substantial involvement in the process. As one noted:

> There are capital equipment items I'd like to see the hospital buy, but they can't afford it right now. I understand the reasons right now, and I can accept those. I think the thing that makes that work well is that in the various areas where physicians are directly concerned, there's adequate physician involvement in the budget-making process. So the doctors are involved in establishing priorities, and they recognize this.

Scripps Memorial Hospital

Scripps has not had any major staff cutbacks in recent years. As reflected in the comments of the respondents, they monitor physician utilization carefully:

> People understand that there's fixed reimbursement now, and I think they're sensitive to that issue. They understand that if the hospital loses money and goes under, they won't have a place to work. I don't think that most people really want to abuse the health care system. You can say to them, why is this patient still here, what is going on? If they really don't have an excuse, by and large they're embarrassed and they'll discharge the patient. . . . The hospital has absolutely never put any pressure on anyone to get a patient out of the hospital except through me [the utilization coordinator], and I won't do it. . . . I won't do it unless I think somebody's really abusing the system. . . . When I have a problem, I use their [the doctors'] patients because I have the ability to issue a denial letter which makes a patient financially responsible for their own stay. Then the patient will become annoyed at the physician, and the physician will discharge the patient. It works reasonably well.

Sutter Health

Sutter attempts to promote effective utilization of resources primarily through the development of their "continuum of care" concept. They

use discharge and home care coordinators to facilitate transfer of hospital patients to intermediate care facilities that are owned by the system,
but there is no direct pressure on physicians. As one notes: "I have to
say that Sutter has . . . never forced me to discharge before I was ready.
No one has ever hassled me over how to take care of somebody personally."

The hospital also relies on physician involvement in budgeting and
finance committees. Like many of the study sites, Sutter is actively
working to develop better cost-accounting practices. The following comments of one physician highlight this concern:

> We are just now getting a cost-accounting system in place so that
> we can get to what our actual costs are. We are dealing with
> charges and trying to guess what the cost is as a percentage of
> charges. As soon as that cost-accounting system is in there, I hope
> to get a system of some kind established so that we can put the two
> together and come up with who might be the bad apples in the
> practice bunch. . . . I looked at some of those things some time ago
> and most of them are typical. I find that most of the patients were
> nursing home patients that came in here after being in nursing
> homes several months. They would come in here and have six
> consultants spend $100,000 and die. Of course, they were all out-
> liers as far as the cost is concerned, but what are you going to do
> about it?

In regard to malpractice, physicians are able to obtain a 10-percent
premium discount if they attend hospital-run risk management educational sessions. The hospitals also provide supplementary coverage for
obstetricians when they treat medically indigent patients.

Tucson Medical Center

Tucson Medical Center had no major staff layoffs, although approximately 90 employees took advantage of an early retirement program.
Some of the things management has done are reflected in the following
comments:

> We've got the highest FTE in the country. You sit down and com-
> pare us with a Baylor or a NKC or a Baptist Memphis, and we're
> high. We're just simply out of the ball park. Somebody else is
> delivering care at fewer FTEs than we are. . . . So we've still got to
> cut. So several years ago, we brought in the Travenol Baxter VIP
> program. . . . That was an attempt with a data base to put a cost
> accountant and a nurse, a doctor, and some other people together
> to take a look at overall care instead of looking at individual pieces.
> . . . We also brought in a management engineering person and put

him on our payroll part-time. . . . VHA is now revving up to do more of that in a different way with [a consulting firm], I believe, and I'm counting on that as another means by which the key players could come together and make some decisions about how we can make some of these adjustments. But I've got to tell you that we have a lot to go through yet because we are out of line in that respect.

Tucson also places heavy emphasis on controlling physician utilization, as indicated by the following physician's remarks:

We're very aware of cost containment. They make us very aware of it. They try to do as much as they can without compromising the quality of care.

Some physicians believe even more can be done. As one noted:

In my opinion they aren't doing enough to address cost containment, but it becomes a very difficult issue. It's potentially divisive, and it may be that they've taken a progressive intelligent approach, but ultimately we're going to have to do more to get things under better control. There are some physicians who, either because of their interests or knowledge, are pretty well attuned to it. There are others where it's almost a blatant disregard, and eventually those are guys that are going to have a change. I don't see the medical staff taking a real strong position on that. I believe that medical staff leadership will support the hospital, but I believe that the medical staff doesn't have a vehicle for that; we don't have the numbers for that. We'd be using the hospital administration to generate the numbers.

TMC requires each physician to have a minimum of $1 million of malpractice coverage. They have umbrella coverage for their high admitters. They are having some problems getting obstetricians to take on-call coverage and neurosurgeons to provide trauma services. The hospital is working hard to get tort reform at the state level.

West Allis Memorial

West Allis is the only hospital in its area that has not had a major layoff or cutback. They work actively with their physicians in containing costs on a daily basis. As an example, the orthopedics department agreed to standardize all equipment used in order to obtain cost savings. The hospital also monitors nurse staffing on an hourly basis, taking into account patient needs.

CONCLUDING OBSERVATIONS AND GUIDELINES

For the most part, hospital efforts to contain costs have not caused major conflicts with physicians. This is due primarily to physician involvement in the decision-making process and to an agreed-upon understanding that to the extent possible, cost-containment efforts will be focused on activities not directly affecting patient care. Rather than worrying obsessively about cutting costs, the study sites have focused their major energy on working more cooperatively with their physicians in expanding revenue sources and market share. At the same time, most sites are engaged in continuing education of physicians regarding cost-effective medical practices and have emphasized strong physician-controlled utilization review programs. In general, the experiences of the ten sites suggest the following cost-containment guidelines:

1. Cost-containment activities need to have heavy physician involvement and, where appropriate, control.

2. Cost-containment efforts should, at least initially, be centered on those areas not directly affecting patient care.

3. Every effort should be made to demonstrate the linkage between cost-effective utilization resources and quality of care (Eisenberg 1986). As will be discussed in Chapter 15, utilization review activities should be linked to the institution's overall risk management, quality assurance, and quality improvement process.

4. Ongoing education of physicians regarding cost-effective practices is required.

5. Cost-containment efforts must be supplemented by programs meeting community needs, which also enhance hospital and physician revenues and market share.

REFERENCE

Eisenberg, J. M. 1986. *Doctors' Decisions and the Cost of Medical Care.* Ann Arbor, MI: Health Administration Press.

CHAPTER 14

Nurse-Physician Relationships

The most surprising finding of the study was the pervasiveness of conflict between nurses and physicians. Nurse-physician tensions were frequently mentioned at eight of the ten sites. The major causes were

1. changes occurring within the nursing profession as reflected in changes in nursing practice
2. an acute shortage of nurses
3. economic and related pressures on physicians resulting in abusive behavior on the patient floors

Each of these causes is examined below along with the approaches which the sites used to deal with the problems.

CHANGES IN THE NURSING PROFESSION AND NURSING PRACTICE

The effects of the increasing professionalization of nursing (for example, longer periods of formal education) are beginning to be felt on the patient floors. Nurses are justifiably claiming the need for greater autonomy and participation in patient care decisions associated with the increased responsibility and accountability for taking care of more acutely ill patients (Aiken 1982). Nurses are also demanding a larger voice in hospitalwide decision making. These "changes within change" interact with the forces described in earlier chapters to create additional strain on the hospital-physician relationship. While they require adjustments on the part of hospital executives, the changes are being felt most acutely by physicians. This is particularly the case for older physicians who have a more traditional view of nurses and nursing practice. The situation is best captured by the comments of several Providence physicians. As one noted:

> I think, as you probably know, doctors like to be the ones that come and have the nurses jump to attention and have everything ready for each doctor and give a quick rundown on what's going on so that he can sign his signature and walk out. There's that "king" aspect that doctors have to deal with. I think the nurses in the last year have become much more independent and want to become more involved in the care-taking process. So they have learned a lot more and have become more involved with patient care, particularly in the ICU and coronary care units. I am sure many of those nurses are equal to, if not better than, some doctors, particularly in emergency situations. On the regular floor, there has been a feeling that the nurses are not so involved with patient care as they are more occupied with administration. As a result you walk on the floor and it's hard to find charts and hard to find nurses. It's hard to document things on the charts. This has been a really sore spot. The nurses have added so much unimportant material to the chart as far as we [the doctors] are concerned. I know it's important to them in terms of nursing care. But, you know, how many times a patient has a bowel movement and how many times they get a back rub . . . is really nice, but it makes it difficult when you approach the charts when all you want to know is what you've written for progress notes or lab reports and you don't want to go through all the other stuff. So the charts have been encumbered and the doctors have gotten upset, and there have been many meetings with the medical records committee to change that. . . . But I know that there is not that genuine warm feeling between doctors and nurses that existed in the past.

Another physician commented:

> It seems to me that the nursing bureaucracy has gotten so large that it's difficult to cut through it and resolve problems having to do with the paperwork and charting of records. Nurses are so burdened with administrative and management duties that there doesn't seem to be any time left for patient care. Also, there is an attitude problem in which many nurses, particularly younger nurses, are so concerned with professional autonomy and not being subjugated to physicians that it can lead to competitive situations that can be detrimental to patient care. I'm sounding like an old fogy suggesting that they should always follow the beck and

call of the doctor and say, "Good morning, sir" on the rounds and do the charts. I really don't feel that way because I'm very much in favor of a collegial relationship between physicians and nurses. But some nurses carry their professional end to an extreme. And to some extent, it may get all caught up in women's rights as well as professional concerns. And the nursing administration has developed such a hierarchy that it's hard to cut through that and establish effective communications.

A third physician commented:

So far, all of the nurses concerned with their paperwork hasn't resulted in poor patient care. And it won't. And it hasn't resulted in poor quality anywhere. What it has resulted in is that the physician is downgraded in his own eyes and in how he interacts. He's not catered to anymore. When you go on the floor, the nurse doesn't come with your charts and say, "I'll go around with you and write everything down that you tell me to." Those days are gone. They don't do that anymore. But there's a lot of doctors who think they should.

In response, the hospital has appointed a patient care committee composed of both nurses and physicians to work through the issues. They have also mounted an educational campaign with physicians, emphasizing that the changes in nursing organization and practice will enable them to recruit and retain the most qualified nurses.

Other sites faced similar challenges as Providence, although without a competing hospital that encouraged more traditional relationships. Five of the ten sites used nurse-physician liaison committees to deal with conflict issues. Another (McAuley) recently completed a major reorganization of its nursing service along the lines of a nursing group practice organization, resulting in greater nursing autonomy.

THE NURSING SHORTAGE

In varying degrees almost all hospitals faced a shortage of nurses in one or more areas. This raised a number of issues related to the decision-making process for approaching the shortage, and physician and nursing roles in this process. The situation at Crouse-Irving Memorial is captured by two physicians' comments. One noted:

The problem with the nursing shortage here is severe. . . . We have about 100 beds closed. I think the medical staff has done something to make that better. We suggested the idea of a tuition program that reimburses nurses if they work here.

. . . But physicians are not a great bunch of people as far as relationships with nurses. I don't know what the problem is with this issue. But they make the life of some of the nurses miserable. And if I were a nurse, there's no way that I would work here. And it's probably true for any hospital. And it's not only in the high tension places like the operating room, but it's just very difficult for nurses overall. I think what's happening is that the nurses are moving into jobs that are 9 to 5, where they don't have to work terrible shifts and on weekends. For instance, the new surgery center opened last year down the street. About half the nurses from the OR went down there. And I don't blame them. I mean I would do that, too. You know, they work eight hours a day, five days a week, and it's terrific. They don't have the problems. They want to raise their families, and they can do this. They don't have as much physician abuse there. There's a problem no matter what anybody told you. . . . I used to think it was only the older people. But it isn't. I can tell you in two years as president of the medical staff, I had more problems with younger physicians than older physicians.

A second physician noted:

I think nursing administration makes decisions which the medical staff should be given more say about. This came up at our last executive committee meeting . . . in an interesting kind of way. The new president came and talked about issues like the coronary care unit. . . . The former chief of surgery got up and said it was very much needed. He pointed out that we make decisions in the intensive care unit that have grave implications for the medical staff. We don't have enough say about those. (The V.P. for nursing was sitting there, and I think she got the message.) So they're going to have this committee. I don't think we [the physicians] have enough say about some of the nursing decisions that are made at the moment. . . . For example, with the shortage of nurses in the intensive care and coronary care units, they decided to combine the units. Now that was not discussed with anybody. . . . So I called [the vice president for nursing] and said, "What's going on?" "Oh," she said, "We're not planning to do it. We're just studying options." I said, "Well, I don't think you ought to study that one because we're not going to do it." . . . But, you see, they were planning to do it, and they should have talked with us first. There's no use planning an option if it's unacceptable with the medical staff. Now they would not have implemented it, I don't think, without our say. We would have said no. But that creates communication problems.

Lexington, like Crouse-Irving Memorial and several other sites, had also closed beds because of a nurse shortage. Lexington's problem was compounded by a two-year vacancy in the nursing director position resulting in decreased morale. The hospital responded to the situation with a six-point plan:

1. developing a physician-nurse liaison committee to do more joint problem solving (the most vocal physicians were placed on the committee)

2. surveying nurses who had left to find out what the problems were

3. forming their own pool of nurses loyal to the hospital

4. downsizing their units to help recruit more nurses

5. obtaining greater physician involvement in in-service education of nurses, for example, instituting a mandatory physical assessment course

6. initiating joint physician-nurse rounds

At West Allis, the approach is to ensure that no nurses lose their job as a result of decreased occupancy. If necessary, jobs are shared and nursing skills made available in other parts of the hospital.

PHYSICIAN STRESS

Many physicians are experiencing increasing stress as they attempt to deal with the growing difficulties of practicing medicine. In some sites, this was reflected in an increased incidence of verbal and physical abuse of nurses and sexual harassment. The situation at one hospital is typical of the problem. A physician who, in the words of a colleague, "ate nurses for breakfast" became particularly abusive with a nurse. The chief of staff took the situation to administration for counseling and advice. They appointed an ad hoc task force to look into the issue. The task force sanctioned the physician and suggested he receive psychiatric counseling, which he agreed to. It was reported as "a great morale builder for the nurses." The hospital believes it needs to be tough with such physicians and send a clear message that "you don't abuse our nursing staff." A similar approach is expressed by the vice president for patient care at another hospital:

> When we have real paranoid physicians, you have to decide on the course you are going to take. When it's a nursing-physician issue

and I feel really strong about it, the upper-level administration has been responsive in helping to sort things out. We recognize that physicians still need to grandstand, make major speeches, the kind of soapbox stuff, and then once they get past all of that, you can usually work out what the key gut issue is. We sometimes take direct hits and do not respond with anger at the moment. But we follow up and let them know that this kind of behavior will not be tolerated.

BEST PRACTICES

Collectively, a number of approaches are being used by the sites to develop better nurse-physician relationships:

1. Establish joint nurse-physician liaison committees with an equal number of nurses and physicians to deal with problem issues. At Leonard Morse, such a committee is cochaired by a physician and a nurse. They try to limit the issues to patient care concerns. They find they need a period of time to build trust before tackling more volatile issues. All members contribute to the agenda. As a result of the committee's work, there has been growing support for nursing from physicians.

2. Establish a nursing futures task force. Among the issues being addressed in such a task force at Scripps are patient scheduling, information systems, the integration of patient and physician satisfaction data into the quality assurance process, developing a fast-track career ladder that will help in recruiting more experienced nurses, and establishing a technology review committee.

3. Initiate a nursing liaison person for every major clinical department head. The function of the liaison person is to work directly with the department head on improving communication and dealing with problems.

4. Have nurses present at all key medical staff meetings and, in turn, have physicians present at all key nursing committee meetings.

5. Institute a system of "dyad doctors," developed at Tucson Medical Center. These are high-admitting physicians who work well with nurses and have the respect of their physician colleagues. They are used by nursing to deal with problem physicians.

6. Develop a system of service facilitator groups, like Tucson Medical Center. These groups are made up of doctors, nurses, other

health professionals, and administrative staff involved with a given service. Their job is to brainstorm new ideas and find ways of providing the service in a more cost-effective manner. In the process, operating problems that develop between doctors and nurses are addressed.

7. Develop a speakers' bureau using a physician-nurse team. This not only presents a favorable external teamwork image to the public but also serves as a powerful internal symbol to physicians and nurses.

8. Develop communication protocols for dealing with nursing issues and problems.

9. Use focus groups with outside facilitators to address some of the more problematic issues. The focus group format is used to surface hidden conflicts and generate positive approaches.

Given the current trends emphasizing more cost-effective patient care practices, it is clear that nursing will play an expanded role and will demand more of a joint partnership with physicians. Among other things, this will require a greater amount of joint training of physicians and nurses in management skills, including coordination, negotiation, problem solving, and leadership approaches. In particular, medical staff and nursing staff leadership will need to work together to set the appropriate tone for the relationship and advance mutual interests. If the experiences of the present sites are any guide, it is unlikely that hospitals and physicians will be able to make much progress in the 1990s without active and ongoing nursing involvement, support, and leadership.

REFERENCE

Aiken, L., Ed. 1982. *Nursing in the 1980s: Crises, Opportunities, Challenges.* Philadelphia: J. B. Lippincott.

CHAPTER 15

Quality Improvement

Chapter 13 discussed the continued pressure on hospitals and physicians for cost containment and fiscal accountability. This chapter examines what the study sites are doing to respond to the growing pressures for clinical accountability. These pressures will grow as advances in health services research make it more possible to measure patient outcomes (Blumberg 1986), assess medical effectiveness (Brook and Lohr 1985), and develop practice guidelines (Roper et al. 1988). The challenge lies in incorporating the advances in research into everyday practices that can be used to evaluate, monitor, and continuously improve the quality of patient care (Berwick 1989).

The study sites were involved in two major sets of activities related to quality improvement: the determination of privileges/review of credentials and quality assurance and assessment. Each is discussed below.

PRIVILEGES AND CREDENTIALS

Reviewing credentials and determining privileges was one of the most frequently mentioned problems noted by all sites. Each had at least one discipline problem during the most recent year, ranging from substance abuse to questionable practices to disruptive behavior. While a couple of these involved lawsuits, in no case did the problems result in a hospital-physician battle, nor did they have a significant effect on other issues facing the hospital and the medical staff. This was primarily due to the strong medical staff leadership and management-physician relationships that existed, as described in previous chapters (see, in particular, Chapters 5 through 9).

Overall, nine of the ten sites felt that they had good to strong credentialing programs; only one cited "some problems." Several, however, indicated that they felt they could be doing an even better job, particularly in speeding up the length of time between the receipt of the application and a decision (in some sites this took over four months). In order to address this problem, some sites developed a one-page preapplication screening questionnaire. One site, Crouse-Irving Memorial, did community-wide credentialing with other hospitals in the area, working through a network of medical directors from each of the hospitals. Tucson Medical Center was considering doing the same. In general, most felt that they did a better job of initial credentialing than of recredentialing and disciplining. As expressed by one board member:

> Yes, it [the review process] works. But I personally don't think it is severe enough. I think you have the fox guarding the chicken house to a degree. I think it is only because certain of these physicians are tough enough to stand up to their brother and say, you know that's wrong . . . that makes it work.

The usual process of review is shown in Figure 15.1. It is highly decentralized: the initial review is done by the individual clinical departments, which then forward the recommendations to the credentials committee. This committee reviews the department's recommendations and ensures that the candidate meets any additional hospitalwide criteria and considerations. It is then passed on to the medical executive committee for approval. From here the recommendations go to the hospital board for final review and approval. Three of the ten hospitals were assisted in this process by a full-time attorney. Most sites reported doing a much more thorough job of investigating candidates' backgrounds than they had done previously.

Several sites have strengthened the interaction between the hospital board and the medical executive committee. Sutter has a four-member board medical policy committee that reviews decisions based on a written report and full documentation provided by the medical executive committee. Tucson has a professional affairs board committee composed of board members and medical executive committee members who review the final recommendations. In a couple of sites (for example, Providence and Scripps), the board has overturned medical executive committee considerations. These decisions did not cause ongoing disagreement because in both cases the parties involved were alerted in advance that there might be a problem and the reasons were well articulated. The "prior informing" was mutual, with both the medical staff executive committee alerting the board of potential developing problems

Figure 15.1   Typical Privileges and Credentials Review Process

Clinical Departmental Review	$\rightarrow$	Credentials Committee	$\rightarrow$	Medical Staff Executive Committee	$\rightarrow$	Hospital Board

and the board alerting the medical executive committee based on the evidence the board had at the time. The joint conference committee was generally used to resolve any lingering disagreements.

At least five of the sites used quality assurance performance profile data in making recredentialing decisions. Several sites were beginning to evaluate physician efficiency in use of resources as a criterion for reappointment. Others were also taking into account how well the individual works with others and ethical considerations.

Perhaps the most elaborate credentialing system was that used by the internal medicine department at McAuley. They assigned points based on such criteria as quality of recommendations, personal interview, evaluation by the medical staff, completion of boards, publications, and rank in medical school. Applications go into a pool, and the best people are selected out each year.

Impaired physicians were recognized by all sites as an issue requiring ongoing attention. Five of the ten sites had their own impaired physician committee, while the remaining five worked closely with the local medical society. Most sites were prompt in taking actions when problems came to a head. A typical situation is described below:

> We just had one of the physicians in our group being investigated. He was seen on the unit a couple of times looking drunk. The quality of his care has certainly fallen off. This week he had three notices. We called him in on Friday and talked about it. The impaired physician committee has called him in now. And they met with me and talked to me about ways to try and help him out. We have arranged to have some of his friends meet with him and deal with him on the committee and try and get him to see that he needs some help. His patients are being monitored much more closely. All of the unit directors have been notified to look after them. Frankly, today, I just changed the on-call schedule so he can't have any on-calls.

QUALITY ASSURANCE AND IMPROVEMENT

All sites recognized the need for improving and upgrading their quality assurance and assessment programs. Quality assurance was evaluated as good to strong in eight of the ten sites and at least average in the remaining two. Six of the ten sites had developed computerized quality assurance systems including physician performance profiles. As previously mentioned, five of the sites explicitly use such data in reviewing physicians for reappointment; most of the others planned to do so once their systems were operating. Almost all sites were working

1. to better integrate quality assurance data and activities with utilization review and risk management data and activities
2. to better integrate medical staff quality assurance with hospital-wide quality assurance
3. to improve the information flow to the board and strengthen the board's involvement in the process

Two sites have recently initiated hospitalwide total quality improvement programs based on industrial quality control principles and practices (Deming 1981). These sites face the additional challenge of integrating traditional quality assurance activities into the new total quality improvement approach. Sites with medical directors felt the position was of great assistance in helping to deal with these issues. Some sites had been able to lower their malpractice insurance premiums since improving their quality assurance process.

Among the major obstacles faced by each site were

1. the increased resources, particularly staffing, required to do more intensive review
2. convincing physicians that the main purpose of the increased quality assurance activities was education and improvement, not punishment
3. dealing with the issue of confidentiality in protecting physicians who served on quality assurance review committees
4. convincing some physicians that the activities were more than window dressing

The approaches of each site are highlighted below.

Crouse-Irving Memorial Hospital

In New York State a list of defined critical incidents (patient care mishaps) must be reported to the commissioner of health. The commissioner's office, in turn, sends letters to hospital board members informing them of these incidents. The state also specifies various criteria for each hospital's quality assurance plan. Crouse-Irving Memorial recently developed a new plan to meet these criteria. The plan integrates both medical staff and hospitalwide quality assurance and risk management activities and is coordinated by the medical director, who works with an overall committee of the board. The board committee members are selected from trustees, medical staff, ancillary professional groups, administration, and nursing. The committee meets quarterly and provides a quarterly report to all trustees. It uses the Commission on Professional and Hospital Activities (CPHA) data for baseline comparison purposes. The hospital was recently reaccredited by the Joint Commission with only one Type I recommendation. The hospital's emphasis on quality is reflected in the following physician's remarks:

> I guess the biggest thing that I find different at this hospital than some others I'm familiar with is that, at least in my mind, the first interest here is on quality rather than the bottom line. . . . They try to provide the best quality equipment, the best quality physical plant, and the best quality medical staff. I guess that is what impresses me most about this hospital over others. I hope that isn't changing but . . . times are tough.

Although time consuming, the importance of quality assurance committee work is expressed in the following physician's comments:

> For the first time, I think we have physicians who realize how important this work is. I think we took it very lightly at first. But I think they realize how important it is because in this state it is required that you have a quality assurance committee (which we do) and it has to have teeth. That is, it looks at these issues and if we think a particular individual is way offbase, he is told that this will go in his permanent file and the state has access to that. So it has a great implication for the individual's career and livelihood. You know it is important committee, but I think it has been very effective; it has been very fair.

Leonard Morse Hospital

Massachusetts also has a number of patient care assessment requirements including a patient care assessment committee. The committee at Leonard Morse is composed of a board member, the hospital CEO, the president of the staff, the vice president for nursing, and other physician and nursing representatives. The first level of peer review is within each medical department. These findings are then communicated to the quality assessment committee, which in turn forwards them to the patient care assessment committee. The process is described as "working well," with improved accountability being one of the rewards. One problem is that the list of state-required patient complaints that must be reported turns out to be, in the words of one, "mostly garbage." This has been a source of frustration to many physicians, which in turn makes the quality assessment coordinator's job more difficult. She has, however, received the support of key physicians. The hospital has a strong utilization review program, is beginning to computerize quality assurance data, and has developed a system for evaluating patient satisfaction.

Lexington Medical Center

Lexington's process of quality assurance and assessment is similar to many of the other sites. They have a strong quality assurance director, who is assisted by a part-time medical director. They regularly send staff to ongoing quality assurance programs. They have computerized some of their data and are beginning to look at practice trends. The data are being used in recredentialing decisions.

McAuley Health Center

McAuley has integrated its quality assurance, utilization review, and risk management functions. They are all overseen by a full-time physician who serves as vice president for quality. As previously noted, they have also initiated a total quality improvement management process, which is also overseen by the vice president for quality. Physicians are closely involved in this process, and a number of them have received formal training in industrial quality control techniques. Some of these physicians are beginning to teach classes to others, including the office staffs of some physicians in private practice.

The quality assurance data at McAuley are computerized; they are used in recredentialing and are beginning to be used for comparison with national norms (including cost norms). Despite the progress that has been made, most agree that the departments need to spend much more time on quality assurance activities.

North Monroe Hospital

North Monroe has a fairly standard quality assurance process that is basically designed to meet Joint Commission criteria. They have the usual committees and do the usual chart reviews. Most respondents indicated the need to get the physicians more involved in the process. Some consideration was also being given to adopting an overall, total quality improvement approach. The philosophy behind this was best expressed by one executive:

> My philosophy is that everyone in the entire hospital is important to providing quality and I'll use two examples. The housekeeper probably sees the patient more than anyone else except the RN or the LPN taking care of the patient. The RN can provide quality service, be pleasant, efficient, and that housekeeper can come in and clean the room, empty the trash, have a negative attitude, and the patient and family will remember that. A dietary aide that delivers the tray and does such a small thing as rolling the tray over to the patient rather then just dropping it and leaving it is showing quality. The patient may not have any family there, may have to call the nurse to come in to roll the table over to the bed, and it can leave a negative impression. So everyone becomes a part of the critical process of quality. Who can solve better the problems of the patients and the hospital than the people who are at the grass roots?

Providence Medical Center

Providence has a patient care review department that coordinates a number of subcommittees, including a medical quality assessment committee, a surgical quality assessment committee, a cardiovascular quality assessment committee, and a PTCA (percutaneous transluminal coronary angioplasty) quality assessment committee. Twenty-three generic screens are used, involving utilization management, credentials, and infection control among others. Sixty-five percent of the screens are done concurrently while the patient is in the hospital, with the remaining 35 percent taking place after discharge. Patient satisfaction data are also examined. The overall quality assessment committee monitors follow-up and corrective action and reports its findings to the medical executive committee. To assist in the process, the hospital uses the Craddick Medical Management Analysis (MMA) system to develop physician profiles. They have found the system to be resource intensive (requiring nine FTEs) and believe that they are understaffed to properly use it. They are also attempting to identify relevant population base data that can be used to compare with individual physician performance profile data. They feel this is needed before they can begin to convince physicians to change their performance. The hospital is also beginning to initiate some quality assurance activities in its satellite primary care clinics.

Providence's quality assurance process also benefits from being a system member. This evidenced in the following example of an adverse drug reaction:

> We found, for example, one institution that was having a very bad outcome with an anesthesia drug. We were able to alert all of our institutions about the problem before any other kind of alert. We have the ability to transfer information quickly. Here was a case where all of the institutions stopped using it, and it was literally weeks before alerts came out from other sources.

Scripps Memorial Hospital

Scripps believes its quality assurance activities have greatly improved over the last three years. They have a combined quality assurance–utilization review committee that reports directly to the board. The activities of this committee are described as follows:

> My current perception is that it [the committee] functions as a data-monitoring committee. That is, it should verify that the process of gathering the data and dissemination of the data is being done appropriately but should not be involved in disciplinary action. . . . The data are provided to supervisory committees like the medical supervisory and surgical supervisory committees, and those people are asked to make decisions about quality and to take action. So it's basically a watchdog data-gathering committee. . . . But the committee also has the responsibility to oversee the supervisory committees when they are not doing their jobs and rat on them and we have done that. There have been several cases in which we perceive that there has been foot-dragging going on.

Like Providence, Scripps uses the Craddick MMA system, which has resulted in the addition of four FTE staff. At present, everything is screened. The data are used for both educational and disciplinary purposes but have not yet been formally used in recredentialing. It's effectiveness is expressed in the comments of the following physician:

> I'm personally aware of several instances in which physician disciplining has occurred because of information gathered through that system that I think would not have come to light otherwise. So, I think it is an effective way to identify and deal with problems.

The Craddick system is supplemented by a second system, Iameter, which provides severity-adjusted data on overall patterns of care. In addition, the hospital does a special review of trauma care along with six other hospitals in the trauma network. They are also beginning to incorporate service quality indicators as part of their overall review process. The following comments reflect some of the difficulties which the hospital has had in getting the physicians to respond to various components of their overall quality assurance activities:

> Basically, before a few years ago, we had no organized QA [quality assurance] outside of the traditional QA. Wève had the usual growing pains with that. I think that the main stumbling blocks are still physician paranoia, confidentiality, and becoming familiar with a canned system. People have had trouble understanding that this is an outline that you are to modify to take care of your own needs. People have been resistant, mainly out of ignorance. This has been a little tough, but I think it is beginning to work. There is an awful lot of data that we generate, like everybody else. A lot of it is a waste of time, but on the other hand we have learned a lot from it and it is a necessary evil right now.

At present, the surgeons are somewhat more comfortable with the process than the internists. Overall, the hospital is emphasizing the educational value of the process internally (as expressed by one physician, "being a domestic cat") while using it externally to compete for more patients ("being an external tiger").

Sutter Health

At Sutter, the medical staff quality assurance activities and the hospital quality assurance activities are integrated through the medical staff executive committee, and the findings then passed on to the board. For cost reasons a severity-adjustment system was deleted from the 1988 budget, but they plan to incorporate such a system in the near future and will then begin to develop computerized performance profiles. They eventually hope to provide a systemwide quality assurance program. At present, a systemwide policy committee made up of the chiefs of staff of each of the Sutter hospitals meets quarterly to review quality assurance activities. One of the problems they face is that a number of physicians question whether enough support people are available to do the job. As indicated by the following comments, others wonder if it isn't all window dressing:

> But from our [the general internist's] perspective, what is happening right now is a tremendous effort in the way of window dressing. It is not really addressing primary care issues. We feel that some real problems are probably being swept under the rug while a bunch of unreal problems are probably being placed in front of the cannon and shot at.

When asked why this is so, the physician responded:

> I suppose it all boils down to how many knowledgeable people you
> have on your staff who are really equipped intellectually, by train-
> ing, and emotionally to do the job of quality control. There aren't
> many. It is a very small cadre of people, and at this point the
> majority of committee members aren't there yet.

Tucson Medical Center

Tucson Medical Center has an active quality assurance program with
computerized profiles used in the recredentialing process. They have a
quality assurance subcommittee for each major hospital committee.
These committees develop and monitor departmentwide quality indicators, which are then reported to the hospitalwide quality assurance committee, which meets every two weeks. This committee, in turn, reports
to the medical director and the medical executive committee, and quarterly reports are then sent to the board. While some of the physicians
question how much of this is beneficial, others believe it is having a
positive effect. In the words of one:

> I don't think it's strained physician relationships. It has brought
> things out that were just ignored in the past, and I think it is
> working very nicely. I am very much involved with that myself,
> and I have been caught a couple of times myself. Everybody gets
> caught. You know it's not the end of the world; it's not like you're a
> bad doctor because you made a mistake. It's a matter of trying to
> do what's right, and we think maybe you fell through the cracks
> here, what's wrong? Well, nothing's wrong, or, gee, I forgot that.
> You don't have to claim malpractice just because there is a little
> problem here. I understand that, and I will make it better.

They believe that the next step that needs to be taken to "really get
people's attention" is to link quality assurance to risk management. This
is underscored by the following physician's comments:

> Well, I believe vehemently that quality assurance and risk manage-
> ment ought to be the same thing. Physicians don't participate in
> risk management until they have an economic involvement, when
> it's going to cost them dollars, when they are going to gain dollars,
> then they are going to participate. On a personal level our 22-man
> group became self-insured a year ago. . . . I thought we were a
> quality group doing a pretty good job before we started that. I've
> got to tell you that since we started that, every one of us have

changed our practices really dramatically. . . . There are things that we don't do any longer, and there are things that we absolutely insist on now that I believe relate to risk management. It wasn't until it was our risk dollars involved that we really instituted that kind of approach. I believe that when the Tucson Medical Center institutes such a program, then there will be the potential for economic gain by doing a better job of risk management.

West Allis Memorial

West Allis has the usual quality assurance committees and processes. The chief elect heads the quality assurance committee, assisted by a full-time nurse. Considerable emphasis is given to nursing department quality studies. They do not yet use physician data for reappointment but are considering doing so. Medical staff and board committees meet quarterly to review the data and to initiate corrective action as necessary.

SUMMARY AND GUIDELINES

Better quality assurance data and processes are needed for both internal quality improvement and to meet the demands of external purchasers and review agencies. Based on the experience of the ten sites, the following guidelines are suggested:

1. The quality improvement program must meet physician needs and values related to improving the quality of care provided, personal growth, and professional achievement. The primary emphasis should be on the education and improvement aspects of the process rather than sanctions.
2. At the same time, physicians must understand that the quality improvement program is part of an overall accountability process, the results of which are one of the inputs to be used in determining reappointment to the staff.
3. The quality improvement process must be flexible enough so that physicians can experiment with it and make it their own. They should be free to add, delete, or modify criteria based on their own clinical judgment and experience while taking into account the existing scientific literature.
4. The quality improvement program must be adequately funded to generate needed severity-adjusted, computerized data profiles for purposes of making internal and external comparisons.

5. The quality improvement program should have clear channels of accountability. Ideally, a single individual should be charged with overall responsibility for the program (for example, a medical director or vice president for quality).

6. The hospital's governing board should receive at least quarterly reports in sufficient detail to understand the major problem areas and with sufficient understanding so as to be able to evaluate recommended corrective actions and hold relevant parties accountable for implementing those actions.

7. The utilization review and risk management functions and activities should be fully integrated into the quality improvement program. The quality improvement program should also incorporate service quality criteria, including patient-generated satisfaction data.

8. Hospitalwide quality assurance activities should be fully coordinated and integrated with medical staff quality assurance activities as part of the overall quality improvement program.

9. The quality assurance program needs to be fully integrated into any hospitalwide total quality improvement process.

10. As resources and expertise become available, the quality improvement program needs to be extended to include ambulatory care and long-term sites so as to ensure continuous improvement in patient quality across the continuum of care.

REFERENCES

Berwick, D. 1989. "Continuous Improvement as an Ideal in Health Care," *New England Journal of Medicine* 320:53–56.

Blumberg, M. 1986. "Risk-Adjusting Health Care Outcomes: A Methodological Review," *Medical Care Review* 43:351–96.

Brook, R. H., and K. N. Lohr. 1985. "Efficacy, Effectiveness, and Quality: Boundary-Crossing Research," *Medical Care* (May):710–22.

Deming, W. 1981. *Japanese Methods for Productivity and Quality*. Washington, DC: George Washington University.

Roper, W. L., W. Winkenwerder, G. M. Hackbarth, and H. Krakauer. 1988. "Effectiveness in Health Care: An Initiative to Evaluate and Improve Medical Practice," *New England Journal of Medicine* 319:1197–202.

PART IV

Building the Future

CHAPTER 16

Future Scenarios

MAJOR FORCES IN THE FUTURE

Part III (Chapters 10 through 15) illustrated how some of the basic processes discussed in Part II (Chapters 4 through 9) were applied to specific issues facing hospitals and physicians. The present chapter identifies nine major forces likely to shape hospital-physician relationships in the future:

1. payment
2. competition
3. technology
4. demographics
5. health care professionals
6. social morbidity
7. industry composition
8. big business
9. information exchange

These are shown in Table 16.1 and highlighted below.

Payment

The past decade has seen the growth of expenditure limits for the payment of inpatient hospital costs for Medicare patients. Other payers have established similar approaches, primarily reflected in the growth of managed care programs. The 1990s will see these approaches applied to the ambulatory care sector, as reflected in the relative value–based fee schedule proposed by the Physician Payment Commission and the

Table 16.1 Major Forces Affecting the Future of Hospital-Physician
Relationships

Payment
Expenditure targets or caps for provision of all care to defined geographic
groups; minimum mandated benefits; payment based on performance; practice
guidelines

Competition
Based on cost/benefit; quality at different prices; value added; highly intense

Technology
"Consumer friendly" technologies, patient self-diagnosis and self-care; bifurcation between high-tech services concentrated in a few hospitals and low-tech
concentrated in ambulatory settings, patient homes, and at work

Demographics and Attitudes
Aging of the population and "baby boomers." What will they need? What will
they want? What are their values about prolonging life?

Health Care Professionals
Care provided by health care terms; shortages of key health professionals; patients and families active participants

Social Morbidity
Drugs, AIDS; what next?

Industry Composition
Regional and local vertically integrated systems; strategic alliances; hospitals'
and multispecialty groups' implications for continuity of care

Big Business
Push for national health insurance or similar plan to deal with exploding costs
and retiree benefits; large-employer coalitions form to obtain nationwide discounts; emphasis on increasing productivity

Information Exchange
Immediate visual communications involving group users; clinical and financial
networking applications across types and levels of care; computer as the adjunctive brain of the health care professional

likely linkage of the fee schedule with expenditure targets. These incremental steps will eventually lead to the establishment of expenditure
targets for the provision of all care to defined geographic groups. The
only sure way to control health care expenditures is to cap them. The
challenge lies in learning how to do this in a way that takes into account
the health status needs of the population being served, that recognizes
the more cost-effective providers, and that can be efficiently admin-
istered (Shortell 1989). Nonetheless, the general thrust will be in this
direction, particularly given the growing commitment to health services

research focusing on patient care outcomes and medical appropriateness. In the 1990s, hospitals and physicians will increasingly be paid
based on their outcomes and adherence to practice guidelines. Some
suggest that the hospital medical staff may be the "accountability unit"
for such payment (Welch 1989), but given the results of the present
study, the joint physician-hospital organization or some derivative may
be a more likely source.

Competition

In the future hospitals and physicians will have to compete on both price
and quality. The winners will be those that can add value as defined by
consumers and purchasers of care. Those hospital-physician combinations that can provide higher quality of care at a given price or, conversely, can provide a given quality of care at a lower price will attract
more patients. Hospitals and physicians must recognize that the most
important perception of quality will be those used by consumers and
purchasers, even though these may differ from those used by hospitals
and physicians. The winning combinations will be those that can differentiate their price-quality attributes relative to competitors (Shortell,
Morrison, and Friedman 1990). It is also important for hospitals and
physicians to recognize that their will be many new types of competitors
in the 1990s as the setting for such competition increasingly shifts away
from the hospital to a wide variety of other settings, ranging from the
home to the workplace to vacation sites.

Technology

The emphasis in the future will be on cost-effective new technologies
that, for the most part, will enable more patients to be treated outside of
the hospital. There will be a bifurcation between high-technology services concentrated in hospitals and low-technology services concentrated
in ambulatory settings, work sites, and patient homes. Great emphasis
will be given to patient access and convenience. The focus will be on
"consumer friendly" technologies that emphasize the patient's understanding and increase the patient's diagnostic capabilities and the patient's ability to adhere to professional advice in implementing treatment
regimens.

Demographics

Two important groups have major implications for hospitals and physicians in the coming decade: the elderly and the current generation of

"baby boomers." The growing percentage of elderly is well docu-mented. What is less well understood is the health care–seeking behav-ior of this population. For the most part, the group 65–74 years of age are healthy and will not be the primary users of chronic or acute care services. Rather, the demand for these services will in the age groups 75–85 and 85 and over. Hospitals and physicians will need to learn to segment the elderly market to appeal to their different needs. The over-85 group will have a large need for long-term care services. Expen-ditures for nursing home costs are expected to increase from the $20 billion reported in 1980 to $129 billion in the year 2000. As for the baby boomers, it is important to remember that in another ten years this cohort will be the "young elderly." It is a generation that has grown up on jogging, swimming, cycling, and stress management. They are likely to be among the healthiest cohorts of elderly we have ever had, and their demand for and use of health care services will be reflected accord-ingly. It is also important to recognize that this generation have grown to become more involved in their care. As such, they will continue to want to play a major role in their diagnosis and treatment and have a major say in how their health care dollars are being spent (Nader 1989).

Health Care Professionals

The trend for more care to be provided by health care teams rather than individual providers will continue to grow. New technology, the shift toward more outpatient care, the development of new health care oc-cupations, and the natural process of professionalizing (Light and Levine 1988; Schneller and Kirkman-Liff 1988) will result in increased conflict. This is likely to be intensified by shortages of nurses, physical therapists, occupational therapists, pharmacists, and related groups. To a great extent, the nature of hospital-physician relationships in the fu-ture will also depend on how well both groups work with a wide range of health care professionals in delivering services to an increasingly discriminating public.

Social Morbidity

The 1980s have seen many hospitals deluged by victims of drugs, alco-hol, and other stresses of modern living. To this has been added the AIDS epidemic, which in 1986 alone cost $80,000 per hospital admission. While it is difficult to predict what the new social morbidity of the 1990s will be, one can be assured that there will be one. Those hospitals and physicians who are incorporating such scenarios currently into their strategic planning efforts will be better prepared to deal with the unknowable and unexpected (Coile 1990). The issue involves developing organizational forms that are flexible enough to deal with surprises.

Industry Composition

The 1990s will see two major developments in continuing industry consolidation: (1) the continued growth of local and regional hospital systems and (2) the growth of multispecialty group practices, which will, in turn, become vertically integrated with the local and regional hospital systems. The percentage of hospitals belonging to systems or alliances is likely to approach 80 percent by the end of the decade (Shortell 1989). But even more significant will be the growth of physician groups (Rundall 1987), with the possibility of 75 percent of physicians practicing in groups by the end of the decade (Coile 1988). Some see these developments as offering an opportunity for vertically integrated regional medical staffs with a central core of specialists surrounded by a broad base of primary care practitioners (Fifer 1987). Whatever the form, the development of vertically integrated systems will challenge hospitals' and physicians' abilities to manage the continuum of care in a coordinated fashion.

Big Business

There is little question that the power in the health care industry is shifting from the professionals to the purchasers (Light and Levine 1988). Given the growing percentage of employers' costs that are represented by health care premiums, several, including Chrysler and Ford, have publicly stated a preference for some form of national health insurance. One can expect to see large employer coalitions forming to obtain nationwide discounts for their employees and small business coalitions forming to share risks. There will be increased scrutiny of what employees are "getting for the employer's money" with development of data systems that match or exceed those of hospitals and physicians. Some hospitals and physicians might be well served to develop joint ventures with local employers to build data bases that can meet the growing demands for accountability.

Information Exchange

In the 1990s computer information-processing technology will become the adjunctive brain of the health care professional and the glue that holds system components together. Those hospitals and physicians that can use the electronic information technology to track patients through the different levels and sites of care will have a distinct advantage. Market, financial, utilization, quality, and patient satisfaction data collected and analyzed on a real-time basis will be essential to compete effectively.

The Bottom Line

The above forces suggest that the 1990s will be a decade of dying and rebirthing. Among the deaths will be

— the end of the independent practicing physician

— the end of the hospital as the comprehensive deliverer of care by itself

— the end of open-ended payment of costs

— the end of professional dominance

Among the new births growing out of the above will be

— the growth of the organizational professional, primarily reflected in the development of medical groups

— the rise of the hospital as the broker of services, primarily reflected in the development of local and regional vertically integrated systems

— the emergence of both clinical and fiscal accountability

— the development of more collaborative professional-consumer relationships

In brief, the 1990s will be the decade of accountability, the decade of affordable, medically appropriate care.

POSSIBLE RESPONSES

Given the above, how will hospitals and physicians respond? Fifer (1987) suggests that the hospital and medical staff organization itself will become more defined in its size and composition with the continuance of the trend toward full-time medical directors and paid department heads. These individuals will exert more line authority over the rest of the staff. The staff itself may be organized less along departmental lines and more along functional lines—for example, the appointment of physicians to various product lines such as cancer centers, women's health centers, wellness centers, and elder care centers. Physicians will be heavily involved in marketing and strategic planning processes as well as in the determination of appropriateness of care and evaluation of outcomes. The influence of primary care physicians will grow as they play an increasingly important role as gatekeepers to the system.

In conducting a number of health-forecasting studies, Coile (1988) also foresees that physicians will have a high level of influence in clinical and strategic decision making. In addition, hospitals are likely to pick their first team of physicians and provide them needed support. Quality will play an increasingly important role: marketing the quality of the staff, targeting buyers that will be selecting hospitals and physicians based on quality, and developing information systems to compare physician performance against peer profiles will become more important. As previously noted, medical groups will continue to grow; smaller groups will merge into larger multispecialty groups; and hospital-based physician groups will be used to staff an increasingly wide range of ambulatory programs. Among the more popular joint venture activities will be medical office buildings, outpatient diagnostic testing centers, freestanding ambulatory centers, hospital-physician networks, and managed care plans. While these represent anticipated happenings, it is also important to consider the underlying emotional tone of the relationship. Stevens, perhaps, best captures the prevailing sentiment when she states:

> Doctor-hospital relations pose problems for the immediate future. There is a sense among doctors and hospital managers that they are antagonists that are engaged in a power struggle which the managers expect to win. However, as in the past, the strongest institutions promise to be those where mutual accommodations can be negotiated (1989, 362).

TEN SITES' EXPERIENCES

What did the study sites themselves have to say about their future? For the most part the study sites were well aware of the future scenarios outlined above, although specific aspects varied from market to market. Five issues were most frequently raised:

1. dealing effectively with the growing world of managed care
2. continuing to explore opportunities for joint ventures and further strengthening existing joint venture activities
3. developing new organizational forms such as PHOs
4. recruiting additional physicians in primary care and selected subspecialty areas
5. continuing to work with physicians in strengthening the economic environment for practicing medicine through a variety of assistance programs

Of the ten sites, three of them felt that their relationship would continue to be strong and would likely face little threat in the coming year or two; five felt that their relationship would continue to be strong but that the strength would, in fact, emerge from being sorely tested; and two sites felt that their relationship may deteriorate somewhat or at least become tougher due to looming problems. It is of interest to note that the three institutions who felt the relationship would grow stronger without facing much of a test all existed in relatively benign environments, while the two who felt their relationship would become tougher existed in less benign environments characterized by a high degree of external regulation. Some of the details are highlighted below.

Crouse-Irving Memorial Hospital

Due to a combination of state regulations, cutbacks in residents' hours, and a shortage of nurses, Crouse-Irving Memorial believes it will be challenging to maintain productive hospital-physician relationships. As expressed by one physician:

> I think the thrust of everybody is to make the relationship more difficult. . . . I can hardly perceive of it [the regulatory environment] as anything other than deliberate. The attempt is to make this a very antagonistic relationship, and I think the challenge for both medical staff and physicians is to remember that we are on the same side. I hope we're going to maintain the relationship we've had, but I would quickly acknowledge that it's going to be harder and harder to do.

The state's efforts to monitor quality of care are seen as unnecessarily prescriptive:

> They'll review the charts, and every patient will have to have a rectal exam, a pelvic exam, an ophthalmologic exam or the reason has to be stated why not on the chart. Now you know that's putting a big burden on the hospital. For example, a 90-year-old lady who's in congestive failure—well, she needs a rectal like she needs a hole in the head most of the time. Patients come into orthopedics 20 years old and healthy for some procedure. He doesn't need a ophthalmologic exam. That's not the hospital's job to do. What they should do is to spend more time improving the quality of primary care outside the hospital so these people get taken care of. They're putting it all on the hospital. . . . The state department is picky and punitive. They shouldn't be so picky, and they should be more education oriented. . . . It hurts us, and it hurts our rela-

tionship with the medical staff. They have to do all of these things. We have to make them do it. And they get mad at us.

The medical director is coordinating the hospital's efforts to deal with cutbacks and residents' hours. So far, a combination of fellows, attendings, and nurse practitioners have been used to fill the gap.

The shortage of nurses is seen as a continuing problem that will be difficult to resolve. Nonemergency surgeries have been cancelled, and emergency room patients requiring surgery often transferred to other hospitals due to lack of nurse staffing for critical care beds. Administration is working on a program to discharge chronic care patients earlier to alternative settings to free up staff and beds. This has resulted in 23 beds opening up, but 55 remain closed.

Leonard Morse Hospital

Leonard Morse also believes the relationship will be tested in the coming years due primarily to Massachusetts's state reimbursement practices, developing managed care issues (see Chapter 11), and the need for changes in the way in which nurses and physicians work with each other (see Chapter 14). Leonard Morse sees the need for changes in a number of areas:

> Well, I think some things are going to have to drastically change. I think the physicians are going to have to operationalize what the regulations are doing to everybody else in the state. The biggest change is going to have to be on length of stay because the hospital cannot afford to be two or three days over the national average. . . . I mean it takes an inordinate amount of nursing resources for every extra patient day, and we can't afford to do that. The nursing practice has to change, and medical practice has to change. . . . The physician has to say to the patient before he puts them in the hospital: "You'll only be staying for a short period of time," because the regulations are forcing us into this. We have to think about how we're going to take care of the patient when they leave before they get into the hospital. And they do not do that now. And if it doesn't happen, then I can't see how this hospital can survive.

Lexington Medical Center

Lexington believes that the existing strong relationship will only get stronger in the coming years. They base this primarily on the momentum gained from recent strategic planning activities that have had full and positive involvement of physicians. In the words of one, "They [the physicians] will see that they get what was promised." Another noted, "We're continuing to mature and grow. We are developing a sense of pride." They believe a test of the relationship will be how developing managed care issues are handled as well as dealing with some surgeons who have an interest in developing their own ambulatory surgery center.

McAuley Health Center

McAuley believes the relationship will continue to be strong but will be severely tested by a number of issues, including the aftermath of the negative experience with the HMO (see Chapter 11), the need to expand volume, the need to recruit additional primary care physicians, and the need to pursue various new practice options such as the possible development of a multispecialty group practice. Their general optimism is expressed in the following comments:

> I think it will improve. I think there will consistently be more and more appreciation that we're in it together. You know, I had a personal and interesting experience. . . . I go to the medical department's business meetings, and I generally sit through the whole meeting. And I was in an OB meeting where there were some very touchy things being discussed, and they decided they wanted to have a vote on whether I should come to that part of the meeting. They asked me to leave and then decided afterwards unanimously that I should attend all of their meetings throughout. You know you have to have that kind of trust level. I'd spent three years trying to build it. I could have lost it all in one morning, but I didn't.

The need for continued flexibility is highlighted in the following comments:

> I think we will involve the new physician channels and . . . the structural relationships. I think we will get to a place of having mutual respect and patience with each other. . . . It's been real helpful to me to understand that there's no endpoint to these relationships . . . that things will continue to happen because of the turbulence within the environment. And in my mind it's kind of like 80-mile-an-hour winds where you change sails and take measures to make sure that your ship will stay intact. There's no difference in our relationships with our physicians. . . . I think we'll have flexibility as an administration, but I think we can also look forward to physician leadership having flexibility for us to involve them in things or to take the actions together. That will

allow us to survive together. At the same time, when there's a 15-mile-an-hour breeze, we can put up the sails and cruise in comfort. We'll do that, too.

North Monroe Hospital

North Monroe generally believed the good relationships that had been developed would continue but expressed some anxiety due to the loss of the trusted CEO. The hospital is expanding services and is sensitive to physician needs. The generally optimistic climate is expressed by one physician in the following:

> I think it will get better. When we first came here there was the North Louisiana Clinic and maybe a few other doctors. And you can see where there might be a tendency to lean towards the clinic type of life, and each of the other doctors felt like they really didn't have much input. And I think it was harder for the administration than at any other time to make all the doctors feel comfortable. I think they did try to be fair to everybody. Now there's more and more people coming on the staff who are either solo or small group people. A lot of doctors are already established in Monroe so there's enough people now that if you have a problem or an issue, you're not alone usually. There's enough people to talk to you, and you can find out if you've got a problem with it. If so, you can present it as a group.

Providence Medical Center

Providence believes its relationship will be strong but will be tested in the near future by a number of events, including the growing amount of charity care that the hospital delivers, the stringent financial environment that it faces, competition from other hospitals, and the ongoing challenges of incorporating a major new medical group. Concerns regarding the charity care issue were expressed by one physician as follows:

> I think you're going to find a struggling institution that's going to take longer than two or three years to get out of any problems that they've got. . . . The institution has a corner on the market of no-pay and low-pay patients. . . . It has so bothered people. It plays such an enormous role in the amount of money coming in and the ability of the hospital to move that it is becoming a crisis. There are physicians who actually openly said, "I admit my DSHS (Department of Social and Health Services) patients at Providence. I admit

my private pay patients to [a competing hospital]." There are people who actually do that. And that's a disaster.

Reacting to some of the financial and competitive pressures, one physician noted:

I think it's going to be tough. I think the outside influences are going to be more divisive. But I think the group practices and the hospital will survive; we're going to figure out how to solve these problems together. So it's going to be painful. But in order to stay in business, we have to minimize these conflicts.

Nonetheless, there is a general consensus that Providence would be up to the task. As expressed by one physician:

Well, I think there are going to be some really good things happening. I think that the first thing is that the hospital is going to be able to clearly outline what their set of challenges are to the physicians. You know, for a long time people have been only guessing on a lot of these and hearing occasional reports. But I think there's going to be a bigger effort to say that these are the roadblocks that we're up against and that these are the challenges that we face. And then I think they are also going to be presenting the information to get physicians more actively involved with the problems. I think there are a lot of problems that physicians will be helping with. I think there are a lot of problems that physicians face, that alternatively the hospital will get more involved in. We're going to have to get even more involved with each other; . . . we can't remain a separate entity as we had once been.

Scripps Memorial Hospital

Although faced by the challenges of the University Medical Center building a satellite hospital only blocks away and the continued intense managed care competition in the area, Scripps foresees a bright future for its relationship. A lot of this stems from the success they recently enjoyed in regard to a joint Scripps-XIMED activity to locate a new physician office building on the hospital's campus. As expressed by one executive:

Well, we'll be tested quite a bit. At the moment, we've built a lot of expectations. It's like announcing you're going to get married and there is a great feeling. But as you get closer and closer to it, you wonder, what am I doing, and then that passes and things get better again. I think firstly, we're at an all-time high and will come down a bit and reality will slip in, and then it will come back up. I say that because it's like two businessmen into starting a business. When you begin to see some of the realities you didn't realize, you grow a little bit more somber. Then you get through that, and you realize that it wasn't so bad.

The ongoing relationship between the hospital and the XIMED physician group is described by one physician as follows:

> Oh, I think we're going to turn into a mutual admiration society. We ought to work hard at allowing each other to flourish within our spheres of influence and be careful not to tread on each other's toes. We need to have enough insights so that we recognize where we can help each other. I see a tremendous opportunity for that where neither party is heavy handed and in creating more of a congenial atmosphere and spirit of cooperation, which will allow both of us to be innovative in terms of new insurance delivery vehicles and letting the doctors prosper. Because if the doctors prosper, the hospital is going to prosper. And it's not necessarily vice versa. I mean the hospital can definitely prosper and the physicians can still take it on the chin, but I don't think that's a long-term viable situation. . . . I think the way to improve the situation is to be forthright with XIMED. It's to be forthright with other situations, where concrete responses are given to questions and answers in a way that the physicians can go away with something in their hands and not just the taste of a good meal or a nice evening.

Perhaps the most buoyant comment came from the following physician:

> I think things are going to be incredibly exciting. This is going to be our best year. I think 1989 is going to be so much fun because finally we're going to be able to talk about the medical office building. We're going to run flags up. We're going to have parties for the board. It's going to be unbelievable. This whole managed care system is going to break wide open, and I think we're going to come out in an incredibly strong relationship because we're going to work and solve that issue together. . . . I think that 1989 is just going to be dynamite. Big year. . . . It will be spectacular.

Sutter Health

Sutter feels the relationship will remain strong but will be tested by the growing economic pressures on physicians, the increased managed care competition with Kaiser, and the challenge of implementing the integrated medical campus concept. Some of the pressures on physicians came to the forefront in a recent strategic planning retreat in which the medical executive committee expressed vigorous frustration at "not being heard and not being able to influence administration." The hospital responded by setting up monthly meetings with medical staff leaders to identify issues and to solve problems, by adding two more physicians to the board, and by initiating educational sessions conducted by physicians to inform board members about the pressures and concerns facing physicians in their practices. One physician indicated that some things will always threaten the staff but that the hospital is trying to be open in their dealings:

> I think that they're proceeding to do what they feel they have to do, and they're doing it as openly as they can in trying to have something for everyone on the staff so that nobody on the staff feels that they're being discriminated against. But, on the other hand, they also recognize that they can't do certain things with everybody on the staff so they're proceeding along that way, too. How the staff responds to that . . . it's just a completely open question.

The hospital's response to managed care and the competition with Kaiser is to try to form a still larger negotiating-delivery unit, as discussed in Chapter 11 and reflected in the following comments:

> I think there will be a narrower group of physicians that will have closer relationships with Sutter and that relationship will benefit both parties. I think the people on the outside will probably be benefited much less so and this may develop into a confrontational issue. I'm assuming when I say this that the whole issue of the Foundation Health Plan has some problems. It has to do with how much you are paid and the medical rates. . . . People are critical of Sutter in this regard. And I think a lot of the relationships between the physicians and Sutter are going to depend on the resolution of the Foundation Health Plan issue.

Tucson Medical Center

Like several of the sites, Tucson Medical Center also believes the relationship will remain strong in the future but will be tested. The economic pressures on physicians, the need to do well in managed care, and the proposed merger with Samaritan Health System in Phoenix were each viewed as ongoing challenges. In regard to outside pressures, one physician commented:

> He [another physician] felt that physicians were being forced to form an alliance with the hospital and that a forced alliance due to external economic pressures could cause the hostility that physicians felt from the external environment to be projected onto their partners, which would be the hospital. He thought that in resolving this difficult kind of situation one would have to rely on the history of trust in working things through that is a characteristic of this institution. The TMC has laid the groundwork for successfully resolving this conflict.

In regard to managed care, another noted:

> I think you're going to see two groups that are going to be the main medical center supporters. One is going to be the Southern Arizona Independent Physicians' [SAIP] group which is supported by the hospital. . . . It's involved in managed care . . . so they're a captive audience. But the people that are involved in that are good people. I think they would have supported TMC anyway. Then a second group is going to be the independent practitioners. Those are the ones that donate money to the hospital. Those are the ones that serve on all the committees. Those are the ones who volunteer their time. . . . That's going to be the other group. . . . Those two groups I think will be positive all the way up. I'm not in SAIP of my choice. But that hasn't hurt my relationship at all. I put 100 percent of my patients in TMC. I think the SAIP is not good in a lot of ways. That's my own personal feelings about joining it. And I have a lot colleagues who have nothing to do with SAIP. But we're totally 100 percent committed to TMC and do more for TMC than the SAIP guys do. . . . So you've got two parallel groups, both just as supportive of one another and the hospital. And it could be that managed care is going to go down the tubes.

TMC recently lost one managed care contract. In response, they have formed an ad hoc committee to deal with the consequences and develop alternatives. A TMC executive also emphasized the importance of timing:

> Timing is everything. It really is. There are many wonderful ideas, but if they're approached at the wrong time, they have negative consequences, and I think that's very, very important [to remember].

West Allis Memorial

West Allis believed their relationships would be tested by a proposed four-hospital affiliation and by continuing managed care pressures. They handled the affiliation issue by involving physicians throughout. It subsequently fell through, to everyone's relief. In regard to managed care, a major concern is that "the medical staff might be less cohesive than in the past if people start signing up with different groups." The hospital-physician joint strategy is to try to seek contacts that benefit both groups.

CONCLUSION

In general, the study sites foresee distinct challenges, and even threats, to their relationship on the one hand; on the other hand, they have confidence in their ability to deal with them. They are facing the future realistically. Some specific steps being taken to further strengthen the relationship are examined in the concluding chapter.

REFERENCES

Coile, R. C., Jr. 1988. "Role of the Physician in VHA Results of a Delphi Survey: Scenario 1995," Health Forecasting Group, Alameda, CA, May 6.
————. 1990. *The New Medicine: Reshaping Medical Practice and Health Care Management.* Rockville, MD: Aspen Publishers.
Fifer, W. R. 1987. "The Hospital Medical Staff of 1997," *Quality Review Bulletin* (June):194–97.
Light, D., and S. Levine. 1988. "The Changing Character of the Medical Profession: A Theoretical Overview," *The Milbank Quarterly* 66(suppl.)10–32.
Nader, R. 1989. "Four Proposals," *Health Management Quarterly* 9(4):20–21.
Rundall, T. G. 1987. "The Organization of Medical Practices: A Population Ecology Perspective," *Medical Care Review* 44(2):375–405.
Schneller, E. S., and B. L. Kirkman-Liff. 1988. "Health Services Management Change in the United States and the British National Health Service," *Journal of Health Administration Education* 6(Summer):593–609.
Shortell, S. M. 1989. "Strategic Choices For All," *Health Management Quarterly* 11(4):26–27.
Shortell, S. M., E. M. Morrison, and B. Friedman. 1990. *Strategic Choices for America's Hospitals: Managing Change in Turbulent Times.* San Francisco: Jossey-Bass.
Stevens, R. 1989. *In Sickness and in Wealth: American Hospitals in the Twentieth Century.* New York: Basic Books.
Welch, W. P. 1989. "Prospective Payment to Medical Staffs: A Proposal," *Health Affairs* (Spring):34–49.

CHAPTER 17

Strengthening the Relationship: The Major Lessons

MAJOR INGREDIENTS FOR EFFECTIVE RELATIONSHIPS

As this book suggests, there is no blueprint, magic bullet, or short cut to develop effective hospital-physician relationships. There is no single factor that dominates. Effective relationships are based on a somewhat complex interaction of history and culture, change and stability, communication, commitment, competence, involvement, trust, and, most of all, hard work and persistence. The major ingredients that cut across most of the sites' experiences, however, were

— importance of history and culture

— management stability

— genuine respect and liking of physicians

— high commitment to honest, open, candid, and frequent communication

— a willingness to share decision making, with early and ongoing physician involvement

— strong physician leadership and physician leadership development programs

— the ability to work together as business partners

— the ability to manage the pace of change

History and Culture

Organizations are shaped by their history, values, and traditions. The study sites, while varying greatly in age (from under 20 years to over 80 years), were no exception. Most institutions had a history and culture of cooperation and collaboration. This ranged from McAuley's having physicians in the hospital from its inception to North Monroe physicians asking the Hospital Corporation of America to build them a hospital.

Despite a generally supportive history and culture, not every site had always enjoyed strong hospital-physician relationships. In fact, most sites had to overcome adversity as reflected in one or more critical incidents, ranging from past crises in CEO leadership to an overall decline in public confidence associated with a sexual assault charge against a key physician. Several sites (North Monroe, West Allis, Sutter, Scripps, Leonard Morse, and Providence) went through turnaround situations. What facilitated these efforts, however, was a desire on the part of both the hospital and its physicians to want to work together, a sense that their destinies were intertwined.

Management Stability

As previously noted (see Chapter 5), most institutions enjoyed considerable management stability, particularly among the top leadership team. This provided the opportunity for developing trust through ongoing communication. Hospitals and physicians could experience each other knowing the other party would follow through on commitments. This was particularly important for physicians, who are typically attached to a local community and hospital for the majority of their professional career, unlike the mobility commonly associated with hospital executives. When physicians know that a management team is going to be in place for a reasonable number of years, then predictability can enter into the relationship. And with predictability comes an increase in trust, and with an increase in trust comes the ability to do more things together, which in turn leads to greater confidence, resulting in a positive upward spiral. In fact, those institutions with the greatest management stability among the study sites experienced fewer problems than those with somewhat less stability. The relatively high turnover rates among hospital CEOs (American College of Healthcare Executives 1988) represent a serious deterrent to the development of effective relationships. To survive high turnover in this position, hospitals need to have strong board and physician leadership.

Respect and Liking for Physicians

As reflected in many of the comments of the executives interviewed, most had a genuine, even enthusiastic, respect and liking for the physicians with whom they worked. These executives chose health care careers because of the opportunity to work with physicians and other health care professionals who help to heal the sick and to manage institutions that help to meet community needs. They built management teams that reflected their philosophy. While they readily expressed the problems, difficulties, and frustrations of working with physicians, they saw these as the challenges of being a health care executive, as part of the job rather than as interruptions in the job.

Communication

The study sites not only recognized the importance of communication, they were actively looking for ways to improve it. They were students of communication, attempting to put into practice the principles discussed in Chapter 6. Perhaps most striking was the willingness to admit their mistakes, to regroup, and to try alternative approaches.

Sharing Decision Making: Promoting Physician Involvement

Most sites used decision-making styles that emphasized the sharing of power, authority, and influence. Given the difficulties facing their hospitals, they recognized not only the merit, but the necessity, of early and ongoing physician involvement. Some executives found it difficult to let go but were reinforced by some early successes and collegial support. The strategic planning process of the institution was the key area for increased physician involvement, and almost all sites could point to certain strategic planning board, management, and medical staff retreats as key milestones in the development of the relationship and breakthroughs in dealing with difficult problems. The effectiveness of this involvement, however, also depended on the strength and maturity of physician leadership.

Strong Physician Leadership

If there is an attribute that perhaps most clearly distinguishes hospitals with effective hospital-physician relationships from those with less effective, it is the strength of physician leadership. The study sites varied somewhat in the strength of their physician leadership, although all were actively working to improve it. As previously noted, most had longer terms of office for their leaders, involved physicians in all aspects of management and governance, made extensive use of internal and external retreats, and targeted younger physicians for future leadership roles. Most had hired, or were thinking of hiring, full-time medical directors and, depending on hospital size, had part-time or full-time section chiefs. Some had programs for physician management/leadership development. Physician leaders had become quite adept at handling credentialing and privileges issues, routine departmental disputes, and basic quality assurance activities. What posed more challenging was addressing the new demands for clinical accountability represented by the emphasis on patient outcomes and practice guidelines and dealing with the new economic challenges of managed care. In the latter regard, many were experimenting with new organizational arrangements that, in turn, demanded new sets of skills and expertise (see Chapters 11 and 12). Most sites recognized the need for a broader scope of medical leadership, one that extended beyond acute inpatient care.

Working Together as Business Partners

As indicated in the previous chapter, almost all sites saw the ability to work together as business partners as key to their future success. They were all moving toward an increased maturity in their economic relationships. At present, most hospitals were meeting physicians more than halfway—being careful not to compete with physician interests while being somewhat flexible in permitting physicians occasionally to develop services that competed with the hospital. The hospitals were playing a long-run game and recognized the need for some physicians to become stronger and more secure before they would be willing to enter into joint initiatives. The strongest partnerships are based on integrating the strengths of each party. At the same time, whenever possible, hospitals were pursuing joint venture opportunities with their physicians. Reinforcing these efforts were a variety of programs to assist physicians in maintaining and increasing their patient base. In order to achieve those objectives, many recognized the possible need for new hospital-physician linkages and were experimenting with a variety of them, ranging from independent practice associations to joint physician-hospital organizations to encouraging the development of multispecialty group practices.

Monitoring the Pace of Change

Among the most difficult challenges faced by the institutions was managing the pace of change. Events seemed to be either moving too fast or not fast enough. Things were, in the words of one, "seldom in sync." Most striking, however, were the attempts of the sites to manage change actively. Overall parameters were established through the strategic planning process. Implementation was guided by standing and ad hoc committees and task forces supplemented by key retreats and selective outside consultation. Sometimes outside events dictated moving faster than the plan originally called for. In these cases, hospitals and physicians drew on the trust and confidence they had with each other to "let it roll" and "shoot in the dark." At other times, when things appeared to be moving too fast and tensions increasing, events would be slowed down. Differences would be aired, and priorities and energy refocused. Several hospitals showed a willingness to admit that they may have been moving too fast or that they made some mistakes, and they had initiated efforts to get things back on track. A major reason why the pace of change could be managed in this fashion is that a foundation of basic trust and goodwill (see Chapter 7) existed coupled with organizational mechanisms for discussing and channeling conflict in positive directions (see Chapter 8).

SOME SURPRISES

A number of challenges facing the sites could be predicted based on current changes in the health care environment: increased competition between hospitals and physicians, continuing pressures for cost containment and performance accountability, and issues involved in working out joint venture activities. The study, however, also revealed a number of surprises: the extent of conflict between nurses and physicians; the relatively large chasm between medical staff leaders and the staff at large; the amount of adversity most sites had overcome; the challenges of involving a different group of younger physicians in leadership roles; and, on the positive side, the strength and growing effectiveness of physician leadership.

A combination of factors has seemed to intensify the usual degree of conflict between nurses and physicians. These factors include the shortage of nurses, changes in the nursing profession and nursing practice, the increased acuity of patients, and economic and related practice stresses on physicians. The results and the approach to these problems were discussed in Chapter 14. What is significant is that each hospital is facing the problem head-on in an active joint problem-solving fashion, rather than ignoring it or smoothing things over on the one hand, or on the other hand, forcing solutions on either party.

While it is generally known that differences exist between the formally elected or appointed physician leaders and the rest of the medical staff, it was somewhat surprising to learn the pervasiveness and extent of the differences in sites that had reputations for strong relationships. Part of this is due to the difficulty of representing an increasingly diverse set of physician interests—despite using the most effective approaches to communication and decision-making involvement. Part is also due to younger physicians' concerns with building their own practice leaving them with little time or interest in serving the hospital. A third factor results from the hospital and the elected medical staff leadership often serving as the visible scapegoat or personification by staff physicians of perceived negative changes occurring in the delivery of health care. The net result is that hospital and physician leaders alike are frequently frustrated in their efforts to bring along the staff at large. Nonetheless, they continue to persist by working to develop stronger department and section chief leadership, greater involvement in decision making—particularly in regard to parallel organization involvement—and continued efforts to target selected younger physicians for leadership roles (see Chapters 5 through 9).

Given the overall strength of the institutions examined, it was also somewhat surprising to learn of events (sometimes within recent years) that if mishandled, could have had a serious impact on the institution. That they were not mishandled is a tribute to both hospital and physician leadership. They serve as a reminder, however, of the relative fragility of the relationship and the importance of constant vigilance and attention.

The challenge of involving younger physicians has been previously noted along with the various approaches to the problem (see Chapter 5). This problem is likely to grow in future years as younger physicians begin to identify more with their single specialty and multispecialty group practice as their primary agent of professional and career socialization rather than the hospital.

What was most surprising about physician leadership was the relative depth of leadership exhibited and the physicians' increasing sophistication to work through their parallel organizations to deal with economic issues. In most places there was a cadre of approximately 6 to 15 physicians who exhibited considerable understanding of the forces shaping health care delivery and their implications for the hospital-physician relationship, and who were willing to undertake substantial responsibility for making the leadership work. The leadership was not simply a function of the current chief of staff. It was buttressed by full-time medical directors, full-time and part-time section chiefs, selected physicians in other hospital management positions, physician leaders of parallel organizations, physician board members, and a strong and continuing physician involvement in the institution's strategic planning process. Time and time again, it was the strength of physician leadership that enabled the institution to deal, in a relatively straightforward and self-contained fashion, with problems that in other hospitals could have erupted into widespread conflict. Even among the study sites, those with the strongest physician leadership were better able to deal with problems than those with relatively less strong leadership. The strength of such leadership was generally a product of a culture of collaboration, a few physicians who played a key mentoring role with colleagues, strong executive leadership that fostered physician involvement, and a supportive, encouraging board.

STUDY SITES' EXPERIENCES

When questioned, almost all of the sites were generally satisfied with the amount of time and degree of energy devoted to nurturing hospital-physician relationships. But, at the same time, many added that "you can never do enough." A McAuley executive:

> I think probably the kind of time is more important to me than how much. I think the kind of time that the service lines are spending is probably necessary. We're doing a better job than we were a year ago in terms of everybody in internal medicine knowing they can call [the service administrator] if they want to complain. . . . We probably need to spend less time doing show and tell. . . . I think we probably have some vacant time. . . . If we don't put a whole lot of the other kind of time in, like going back to the marriage analogy, you can fight, but only if you're spending more time doing other things than you are fighting. And we will fight. That's going to be part of the constraints—we're so tightly bound; we need to do that, too.

A Providence executive:

> I would have more retreats. So they would get to know managers better. I would have opportunities for them to get more of the education of our mission and the hospital's strategy. I would have them have more personal relationships with the administrators and in essence have the administrators spend more time with them. . . . I think we have to make ourselves more available. I think the reason you can't get doctors in here to talk to us is because they're very busy making a living. And as public policy impacts get tighter, they're going to be even busier making a living. Yet we have a mutual product here. We're like a big company, and we can't be separated. . . . So we have this product that we need to have time together to run or administer.

A Providence physician:

> A little more could be done. I'm overall pretty satisfied, but I think a little more could be done. You know, one thing I'm thinking about that's missing is that there isn't cultivation of leadership as a skill. It's kind of assumed that if you're a vocal physician, you are a

leader. But this is not anything you get in medical school. There are natural leaders, and there are people that kind of acquire these skills, and there are some people that need to be trained how to do this. You need to be trained in how to deal with conflict and how to negotiate and how to communicate and all of these kinds of things. We depend so much on the luck of the draw. . . . Perhaps one way to get better relationships is to have either workshops or retreats where the focus is on developing leadership. Unfortunately, physicians, I don't think, want to be bothered with that. They kind of think, "Well, I run an office. I'm on my own. I call the shots. I'm a leader." And the connection hasn't been made as far as effective leadership.

A Tucson executive:

I find myself in the last year having grown away from being as close to the physicians as I want to be, and I'm highly dependent on others. I think that's working fine, but I haven't been able to carve out as much time as I used to, to just roam around the place. And so my own satisfaction there is not real good.

A Scripps physician:

I think what's being done is being done reasonably well, but I don't think enough is being done. Maybe a medical director again is a good example. I think there are areas which the administration should expand into, but they're not. The things that they do, they do well, but they're not doing enough different things.

A Crouse-Irving Memorial executive:

We spend too little time only because we're distracted by the enormous reimbursement problems we have in the state of New York. When you asked me to even participate in this [the study], I thought, well, it's very distracting. You know, you've got everybody on your back; you've got the banker; you've got the bondholders; you've got the state authority. So I probably have to say to you that we spent less time this year than we ever have on the physician relationship.

A West Allis physician noted:

The changing times have increased the pressures. You need to spend more time now.

Among the most frequently mentioned and important plans for further strengthening the relationship were

— continuing attention to communication

— increasing physician involvement and leadership development

— paying increased attention to developing business relationships with physicians
— continuing physician practice assistance
— continuing physician education
— continuing attention to recruiting additional physicians

Continued Emphasis on Communication

The need to give continuous attention to multiple forms of communication was high on the list of all sites. One-on-one and group communication of both verbal and written forms were noted. The need to give more time to in-depth communication and, in particular, to nurse-physician relationship issues was emphasized. A Crouse-Irving Memorial board member:

We had been working on trying to communicate more in writing, not only to the medical staff, but to other staff and even to the community. We try to explain more about our successes as well as our challenges.

A Crouse-Irving Memorial executive:

We're trying to discuss some of the issues that are physician-nursing related. . . . I think we have to work harder next year at getting physicians to look at what they're asking staff to do. What are the real needs in managing that patient?

Crouse-Irving Memorial physician noted:

I think a few of the mechanisms are in place. I think we have a pretty open communication system, but my honest opinion is that we've just been reacting. The pressure is so intense that I'm not sure we've really had the ability to sit back and plan things in terms of how they're going to be five or ten years down the road. We're spending enormous energy to meet the deadlines, to meet the regulatory requirements.

A Providence physician commented:

I would, perhaps, reassess how physicians and hospital administration interact. . . . It feels like two pyramids facing each other. You know, the tips meet somewhere around the executive bay . . . maybe between the medical director and [the CEO], I'm not sure. But I think that is expecting a lot, you know, to have things being processed and dribbled down and have all this stuff come up and meet at these two points. We may have to reassess and have broader contact and involvement.

A Scripps physician commented:

> Effective communication is a day-to-day, ongoing dialogue. . . . I think we need more administrative members showing up in the doctors' lounge, for instance. They need a sense of camaraderie and a sense that we're all in this together. If we don't both survive and help each other, we're all going to die here.

Increased Physician Involvement and Leadership Development

Although all sites already had quite extensive physician involvement in governance and management activities, most believed they needed to do more, particularly in regard to involving younger physicians. During the most recent year, Providence and Sutter added physicians to their advisory and governing boards, respectively. West Allis had extensive physician involvement over many months in deciding whether or not to join a four-hospital network. McAuley, Providence, Scripps, and Sutter had recent key retreats that helped to clarify issues and ensure that the two groups' priorities were largely overlapping and proceeding on track. Scripps participants described their retreat as "a free-flowing discussion about hospital plans, practice enhancement opportunities, and quality assurance." They felt it helped to further open channels of communication. As expressed by one participant, "Although we won't always agree, we all have more to gain by working together rather than separately." McAuley's previously mentioned PHYSICIANS 2000 project has been instrumental in, as expressed by one participant, "bringing backroom issues out on the table for better mutual understanding."

Enhancing the medical director role and increasing physician management skills are also seen as important factors. A Tucson physician commented:

> I think [the medical director role] is excellent. He does a good job and he offers us things that we don't know. . . . He has an awful lot to do, and I'm not sure we couldn't have another medical director. I'm not sure that our staff of the hospital isn't overwhelmed with too many administrative people. . . . I may be wrong, but not in the area of the medical director. I think he's very effective. He's very good at communicating, and he's very knowledgeable about what can and cannot be done . . . but I'm not sure that he isn't drawn about as thin as he can be drawn.

A Providence physician commented:

> I think it would almost be impossible to function without the medical director. . . . I know that it is interesting that we had a medical

director here before . . . who was very effective. . . . For a good-sized hospital to function, it is essential to have a medical director.

A McAuley physician commented on the challenges of moving back and forth between clinical and managerial mindsets:

I think part of whatever modest success I've enjoyed has been that I can sit down and listen and hear the nurses out. I can hear the administrative perspective and listen to my colleagues in this department and just sort of absorb it all and try to come to some reasonable decisions about things. But, there's no way you can always do that. If you're a surgeon, you can't mark out 15 minutes doing aorta resections and do it. It takes some time. One of the hardest things that I've found in the job is shifting from one mode to the other mode. The cardiologists deal with a lot of emergency stuff. I go from this mode of heart stopping, people dying, angry relatives and frustrated house officers, frazzled nurses, and all that. Then, all of a sudden you go into the room, and the administrator wants you to look at these little graphs and charts and blah, blah, blah. That's just a completely different mode, and it's very, very difficult to shift gears, to be in that kind of contemplative committee mode, move back into the cardiac arrest mode, and then shift back again into the committee meeting.

A Sutter executive commented:

We have a plan for future medical staff leaders. We send them to department sessions. I think there has been a recognition by the physicians that they need more help in certain things. I know [a doctor] has an orientation program, and I think they need some more structural skills like how to run a meeting, how you effectively communicate, and that kind of thing.

A North Monroe manager noted:

We work behind the scene with the informal medical staff leaders about the fact that a couple of the new young docs are to be given some leadership roles, either on committees or as officers, to get them involved. And what has happened is that they have done this. They have redesigned our credentials committee so that probably a third of our young docs who have been in practice 2 or 3 years are bouncing over the older docs that have been in practice 15 to 20 years. So we've got both the old and new perspectives. The young docs are picking up some things from the older doctors and vice versa. In order to get our executive committee rearranged this way, they put on a couple of young doctors as secretary of the medical staff, and this year they felt very comfortable putting a young doc on as vice chief of staff. My chief of staff right now is an extremely outstanding, brilliant doctor, good politician, and he really has been an excellent mentor for the chief of staff that will be coming on in January. What I think is essential if you want the hospital momentum to continue is to groom these young guys because they don't know this stuff in med school. They've got to understand the politics. They are naive, and they've got to hear some of these discussions.

Overall, the increased involvement of physicians reflects a shift from egoistic power over others to a more synergic power shared with others. From such involvement, hospitals and physicians may evolve to a form of metaphoric power—the power associated with a shared vision (Kaiser 1990).

Strengthening Business Relationships

At least five of the sites saw strengthening the business relationship with their physicians as key to future success. Some physician organizations were beginning to do their own strategic planning to complement that of the hospital (for example, Scripps and Sutter). All indicated the need for improving everyone's understanding of managed care and strengthening their capabilities to deal with it. A Tucson physician:

> Within the Southern Arizona Independent Physicians, he [a leading physician] had a very clear priority for increasing the number of educational meetings with those physicians who are less involved in general so that they could become more aware of their environment, of the issues that are facing the SAIP, in order to build involvement, participation, and commitment. A second priority he had as president was to develop a consensus on quality in specialized areas such as cardiology. . . . His comment was that the only way you can develop compliance with independent physicians is to have their involvement. While it takes a lot of time, one can only achieve quality effectiveness within the SAIP by having extended involvement from the physicians themselves in terms of quality indicators and quality measures. He spends a lot of time on this commenting that one can never legislate through rules and regulation the enforcement or practice of quality. They have to be economically interdependent. And, they have to establish their own priorities and their own quality indicators through consensus building and acknowledge that it takes a lot of time and effort.

A Leonard Morse board member commented:

In managed care I think the administration is doing a lot of catching up in terms of what our costs are, what our current programs are doing for us, and what is the competitive environment. The trustees are encouraging and financially willing to support the medical staff in terms of coming along to play this game. I think the medical staff is moving slowly in the right direction. I think we got this last HMO thing healed, and then I think maybe the biggest thing that's going to happen in the next year is that the scab will stop coming off. I think everybody is able to talk about it. Although it doesn't mean the same thing to everybody. We don't even have a common language yet for what this does mean. I think there are still a lot of issues about in-hospital managed care versus joint ventures and outside things, and we are really trying to struggle with these issues.

A Leonard Morse physician indicated some of the problems that some physicians have an understanding the ethics of business and economic relationships.

My own view is that sometimes administration is too smart for their own good. I think there's a cultural gap here. Management is taught that as long as it's legal it's OK. But the physician might view that as bad faith. A physician looks at faith. A physician looks at a violation of the spirit of the agreement and not just the agreement itself. . . . The physician can never get over the fact that in a court of law two lawyers can go at each other and afterwards they can have lunch together. That's something they [the physicians] don't understand. So if physicians are in a negotiation and they lose something, they view that as not good and they expect some correction. But management maybe looks at it as a business matter of who can give you the better deal. And this is the same thing for the insurance company. . . . Now it may be ethical in business to say, gee, what's wrong if somebody can give me a better deal, but from a physician's standpoint that's wrong. That's the reason why there is a pervasive feeling among physicians that the insurance people, and sometimes the hospital, are unethical people.

A Tucson physician commented:

I see it [a joint venture involving an imaging center] as being a real turning point for the PHO. As soon as we feel comfortable with where we are with the HMO in terms of being able to manage medical care costs and as soon as we know that the data system that we're getting from the manager truly reflects what's happening within the HMO, we intend to capitate with the HMO for all medical costs. And we'll capitate at a level that will allow us, if we manage well, to have a significant amount of money left over which will belong to the PHO. The PHO will then decide how it's going to use that money. But what we've been doing up until now is we've been taking money from SAIP and from the hospital as seed money for our projects and then borrowing on a line of credit to carry the projects forward. And what we need is an infusion of a significant amount of capital that truly belongs to the PHO that isn't a gift from the hospital or anything else. If we can make that happen, it's going to really take off.

Along with other issues, a Sutter executive highlighted the importance of being able to develop an integrated continuum of care:

I think there are about five factors that will lead to our continued success, and at least a couple of them are involved with the medical staff. One is we need to continue to focus on the operating effectiveness of the hospital. We are going to have to reinvest for the patient care model. We simply cannot go on with the nurse shortage and economic pressures. That will impact on and involve the medical staff. Secondly, we will continue economically advantageous joint ventures with the medical staff because we believe in them and they work for us. Thirdly, we will continue to foster the development of a strong managed care model. That will obviously impact on the medical community. Fourthly, we are evolving into what I've labeled "an integrated health care organization" providing high-quality service and a continuum of care all the way from management and group practices through immediate care centers . . . long-term care, medical equipment, and so forth. That will impact the medical staff in two ways. One, there may be economic opportunities. Two, they will know that we have a committed or controlled patient care capacity that meets our standards of quality. The long-term care venture and the retirement center are examples (even though both are way off economically). We lose money heavily there because it has taken far more resources . . . to bring those facilities up to the standards that are a part of our philosophy.

Continuing Practice Assistance

All sites were involved to varying degrees in physician practice management assistance programs. These typically involved market research to assess physician practice needs and then the development of a portfolio of programs and services to meet those needs, ranging from physician referral services, to office staff management, to development of information systems to better link the physician's office to the hospital. A couple of sites, such as Crouse-Irving Memorial, had standing physician marketing task forces (chaired by the medical director). Other sites, such as Lexington, were developing tailored programs targeted to their most loyal physicians. A North Monroe physician commented:

> I've always thought that marketing can be improved. . . . They'll market the women's stuff, they'll market the rehab center, and they'll market neonatal and ICUs, but there's nothing done in terms of heart surgery.

A Tucson executive commented on the importance of information systems:

> A lot of money is going into management information systems, which we consider to be the heart of our ability to make good decisions and analyze things and tie the doctors in. We've got to find a way to tie that doctor so close to this hospital through the use of that computer and other techniques that he'll think three times before he goes to another hospital. So that's going to be a challenge. And we can do that with capital investment. Can we do it successfully? We've got the authorization to proceed.

A McAuley physician noted:

> One of the things that I've set up is a physician liaison program. I've got people going out and interviewing office managers as well as physicians . . . and trying to identify problem areas. . . . They're also talking to people who refer patients to us. And hopefully we're going to be able to come up with a list of things that we can to do improve services to physicians. We've looked at a number of ways and are continuing to do this . . . a number of ways where we might be able to help the business side of the practice of medicine, including trying to put together a group benefit package that physicians could participate in and looking at whether or not we could do things like payroll and that sort of thing. And then we've also got a group looking at networking information systems with offices, at least initially for the purpose of lab result reporting.

The role that a hospital system can play in fostering a customer-oriented focus is highlighted by one North Monroe physician:

> Again, I suspect that somewhere in Nashville . . . there must be a little training ground for HCA [Hospital Corporation of America] administrators where each administrator spends a great deal of time in a concentration camp learning that the patient is in a hotel

for sick people. Sick people cannot check into the hotel; doctors must put them in the hotel. Keep doctors and sick patients happy. And that is a resounding theme that is not said but certainly echoes throughout for all the administrators to deal with. I think that's probably from the very top down. . . . I've never known HCA to embark on anything where the bottom line was not excellence in patient care. It seems to me that they understand that once excellence in patient care is achieved, then the bottom line takes care of itself.

Continuing Physician Education

All sites indicated they would be giving increased attention to educating physicians about the new economic, ethical, legal, and social realities of health care delivery. In addition to special educational sessions, they planned to use the everyday forms of communication (one-on-one, committees and task forces, and so forth) for such education. They recognized that the best way to get people's attention is to pitch messages to what interests them and affects their everyday life.

Physician Recruitment

A number of sites (McAuley, North Monroe, Tucson Medical Center, and Lexington) planned to strengthen their ability to deal with the future by recruiting additional primary care physicians. They were each working carefully to involve specialists and existing primary care physicians in these efforts. They recognized that the ability to deal effectively with managed care issues would depend in large part on having a strong nucleus of high-quality cost-effective primary care physicians.

One-Year Follow-Up

It is of interest to note that at a follow-up symposium held approximately one year after the initial interviews, seven of nine hospitals participating in the symposium indicated that the relationship had grown even stronger in comparison with the previous year. The other two felt their relationship was about the same. One already had a strong relationship but believed it had failed to make further strides because some medical staff members were beginning to lose confidence in themselves and the hospital as they begin to see their incomes decline. In the second case, the relationship could be described as generally good but strained by state regulation. Their situation a year later was summed up by one as "our successes are matched by our failures."

CONCLUSION

This concluding chapter has summarized some of the major lessons that cut across the experiences of nearly all sites and has highlighted some of the things the sites are doing to further strengthen the relationship for the 1990s. It is important to recognize, however, that what was possible for some was not possible for others. Each was influenced by the constraints and opportunities associated with its environment. For example, Tucson Medical Center, with many of its physicians having appointments at several hospitals, had a much different environment than McAuley, where most of its physicians admitted only to it. Certainly Crouse-Irving Memorial and Leonard Morse, operating in highly regulated states, faced some additional and different problems than the other sites studied. The sites also differed in the type of intensity of competition faced. For example, the intense managed care competition experienced by Tucson Medical Center, Scripps, and Sutter was in stark contrast to that experienced by Lexington, North Monroe, and for that matter, Crouse-Irving Memorial. No hospital in the study matched the charity care responsibilities taken on by Providence. The lessons, guidelines, and best practices associated with the basic building blocks of effective relationships discussed in Chapters 5 through 9 are relevant for all of these situations, but the way in which they are applied and their relative importance at different times will vary. Certainly the special issues discussed in Part III (Chapters 10 through 15), differed from site to site and, as a result, required different problem-solving approaches.

It is also important to recognize that the sites were studied at a defined point in time in their relationship. Having been selected as relatively outstanding examples of effective hospital-physician relationships, most of the sites had advanced to a relatively mature stage. Table 17.1 depicts a simplified stage model of the hospital-physician relationship based on the capabilities and experience of the parties involved. Without discussing each characteristic or requirement, the general point is that executives who find themselves in Stage I infancy relationships have a much different challenge, calling for different skills and approaches, than those in Stage II (adolescence) or Stage III (mature) relationships. It is also important to note that these stages have relatively little to do with the organization's age and do not necessarily follow the sequential path shown. For example, a stressful external event, CEO turnover, or the retirement of some key physician leaders may throw a Stage III mature relationship into a Stage II or even Stage I mode. The key point is the need for CEOs and physician leaders to diagnose the maturity of the relationship relative to the demands of the environment and take the necessary steps to keep it strong and evolving toward ever higher levels of achievement.

Table 17.1 A Stage Model of Hospital-Physician Relationships

Stages	Characteristics	Requirements for Effectiveness

Stage I
Early (infancy)
	Low experience
	Low capabilities
	Low confidence
		Strong culture
		Strong board
		Extensive education
		Develop relationship
		    fundamentals
		High outside
		    consultation
		Some early successes

Stage II
Middle (adolescence)
	Some experience
	Some capabilities
	Moderate confidence
	    but sometimes misplaced
	    sometimes a false
	    confidence
		Understanding board
		Patient administration
		Willingness to
		    experiment
		Ability to accept failure
		Learn from mistakes
		Continued education
		Some trust-builders

State III Late (adult maturity)	High experience High capabilities High confidence	Facilitating board Shared management and governance Build on successes Seek new opportunities Continued education Avoid complacency Some failures

During one of the interviews, a respondent commented, "Life around here is like a three-ring circus." Upon questioning, it was evident that he was not referring to the familiar triad of board, management, and medical staff, but simply to the complexity surrounding modern-day hospital-physician relationships. Upon reflection, it seems that this is as it should be. But it is crucial that one identify the three most important rings. They are the hospital's strategy, structure, and behavioral processes as they influence and are influenced by the hospital's environment. It may be useful to think of the environment as the audience and tent, with the circus being played out in the three rings represented by the hospital's strategy (its goals, and plans for achieving those goals), its structure (arrangement of positions, committees, task forces, and parallel organizations), and its behavioral processes (communication, coordination, decision-making styles, problem solving, conflict resolution, trust building, etc.). Like a good ringmaster, the manager's job is to make sure the activities going on in three rings (the strategizing, the structuring, and the processing) are reasonably complementary and in alignment with each other. The transaction costs (see Chapter 2) must be minimized, and the benefits maximized. They must complement each other for the audience to be pleased. And so it is that hospitals and physicians will need to coordinate their acts and, in the vernacular, get it together for the American public to be pleased.

It is a call for integrated leadership (Joint Commission on Accreditation of Healthcare Organizations 1990) and, ultimately, a new form of health care organization—an organization characterized by joint clinical and fiscal accountability, joint risk and reward, and joint management and governance. As indicated by changes in the United Kingdom and European health care systems (Pettigrew, McKee, and Ferlie 1989), the call is not limited to the United States. It is the infrastructure that will determine how efficiently and effectively Americans receive their care. It is hoped that the experiences shared by the ten sites will assist others in building a stronger infrastructure.

REFERENCES

American College of Healthcare Executives, American Hospital Association, and Heidrick and Struggles. 1988. *CEO Turnover Report.* Chicago: American Hospital Association.

Joint Commission on Accreditation of Healthcare Organizations. 1990. *Leadership Standards.* Chicago, II.

Kaiser, L. 1990. Presentation at Estes Park Institute Conference, "Market Warfare: Hospitals and Physicians in a Competitive Environment," Kona, Hawaii, January 20, 1990.

Pettigrew, A., L. McKee, and E. Ferlie. 1989. "Managing Strategic Service Change in the NHS," *Health Services Management Research* 2(1):20–31.

APPENDIX A

Forms Used for Data Collection

EFFECTIVE HOSPITAL-PHYSICIAN RELATIONSHIP STUDY
INTERVIEW QUESTIONNAIRE

Hospital Name: _____

Person Interviewed: _____

Position: _____

Phone # for Follow-Up: _____

Date: _____

Interview Completed by: _____

1. What distinguishes this hospital from others in the area? What is it particularly known for?

2. How has the hospital's past history and tradition influenced its relationships with its physicians? (Has the hospital historically been specialty dominated, or primary care physician dominated? Has this changed in recent years? Why and what have been the implications?)

3. What principal external factors are placing stress on your hospital's relationships with its physicians (e.g., competition, managed care, regulation, etc.)?

4. How would you describe the current status of Board-Management-Medical Staff relationships at the hospital? (How strong are they? What problems exist? How different is the relationship now from a year ago?)

5. What criteria or indicators do you use to judge the effectiveness of your relationship (e.g., staff recruitment and retention, timeliness of decisions, ability to move ahead with plans, absence of major divisive forces, etc.)?

6. What have been the most significant accomplishments associated with your relationship over the past year or so? (List two or three.)

7. To what do you attribute your success? (If not mentioned, ask about CEO and management's leadership and decision-making style, role of the board, medical staff leadership, hospital culture, physician involvement in hospital governance and management, and the role played by trust, communication, conflict management and managing the change process.)

8. What do you think is the principal basis for *trust* between the hospital and its physicians? Upon what is it based (e.g., past history, experience in working with each other, hospital philosophy, etc.)?

9. With what specific problems or obstacles have you had to deal this past year? (List three or four.)

10. What specific approaches have you used to deal with these issues? What seems to be working, and what isn't working? What are the main committees, groups, or mechanisms you use to manage conflict?

11. How are you currently dealing with the following issues? (How do you handle these issues? How do you resolve disagreements relevant to these issues?) *Have them address each* briefly *and to the point.*

    a. Physician credentialing—new members and renewal of privileges. Open vs. closed staff issues.
    b. Physician disciplining—restriction or revocation of privileges.
    c. Impaired physicians.
    d. Malpractice insurance.
    e. Hospital-physician competition in starting new programs and services—particularly on an ambulatory care basis.
    f. Hospital efforts to contain costs—staff reductions, service deletion, etc.
    g. Exclusivity issues in hospital-physician joint venture relationships.
    h. Improving quality assurance efforts.
    i. Grooming younger physicians for future staff leadership.

12. Is the medical staff primarily viewed as a part of hospital organization, or is it primarily viewed as a separate unit? Why?

13. Are there responsibilities or activities currently performed by the medical staff which could be better performed by another group or unit? If yes, what are these?

14. To what extent do the formally elected physician leaders act effectively in (a) serving physician interests, (b) relating to hospital management, and (c) relating to the board?

15. How would you describe the current level of physician involvement in hospital management and governance? Is it too much, too little, appropriate, inappropriate? (Specifically, ask how physicians are involved in the hospital's strategic planning process.)

16. To what extent do physicians have adequate and appropriate influence over the following issues?

    a. Hospital mission and goals.
    b. The hospital's strategic plan.
    c. Major capital projects.
    d. Acquiring new technology and equipment.
    e. Nurse staffing.

17. How satisfied are you with the time, resources, and energy devoted to nurturing effective hospital-physician relationships at this institution? Is too much time devoted to it, too little, etc.?

18. How do you see hospital-physician relationships at your institution evolving over the next year or so?

19. What are you doing or planning to do to further strengthen the relationship?

20. What other thoughts do you have regarding the issues we've discussed or other points you wish to raise?

THANK PERSON FOR THEIR TIME AND ASK IF IT WOULD BE OKAY TO CALL THEM IN THE FUTURE TO CLARIFY POINTS OR FOLLOW-UP OBSERVATIONS, IF NECESSARY.

ADDITIONAL QUESTIONS TO ASK *EVP for MEDICAL AFFAIRS* (or equivalent), *Physician in charge of QUALITY ASSURANCE* and *Physician in charge of the PARALLEL ORGANIZATION* (e.g., IPA, PPA, joint hospital-physician organization, etc.).

EVP { 1. Please describe your primary roles and responsibilities as the
        _____.

QA {
PO {

       2. In what ways do you relate to (a) the president of the medical staff and (b) the hospital CEO?

QA   3. How does your quality assurance program currently work?
only   What plans do you have to improve it even further?

DOCUMENT SUMMARY FORM

ABSTRACTING BOARD AND MEDICAL STAFF
EXECUTIVE COMMITTEE MINUTES

Site: _____

Date: _____

Type of Document: _____

Date of Document: _____

1. Types of people or positions present at the meeting:

2. Summary of the key issues discussed at the meeting: (UP TO FIVE)

    a.
    b.
    c.
    d.
    e.

3. Issues for which a *formal* vote was taken:

Issue	In Favor	Against	Abstaining
a.			
b.			
c.			
d.			
e.			

4. Do the minutes of this meeting serve as good examples of any of the following? If so, briefly describe how?

    a. *Communication among the relevant parties involved* (either positive or negative)
    b. *Approaches to managing conflict* (either positive or negative)
    c. *Evidence of trust or mistrust among the parties involved*
    d. *Leadership/decision-making style of the parties involved*
    e. *Managing change* (e.g., creating a vision, taking practical first steps, providing ongoing support, etc.)

5. Any other information from this meeting which provides insight into board-hospital-physician relationships at this institution?

HOSPITAL-PHYSICIAN QUESTIONNAIRE

INSTRUCTIONS: Please indicate your degree of agreement or disagreement with each of the statements below. We are interested in your honest, candid opinion of each statement. After completion, please place in the CONFIDENTIAL envelope attached and bring it with you to your interview. Thank you.

Statement	Strongly Agree	Agree	Neither Agree Nor Disagree	Disagree	Strongly Disagree
SECTION A					
1. The hospital gives physicians sufficient autonomy to practice medicine.	5	4	3	2	1
2. The hospital supports the physician's private practice (e.g., physician referral service, practice management assistance, etc.).	5	4	3	2	1
3. The hospital provides the needed personnel to support quality care.	5	4	3	2	1
4. The hospital provides the needed equipment and services to support quality care.	5	4	3	2	1
5. The hospital is careful not to compete with its medical staff.	5	4	3	2	1
6. The hospital administration ensures cost-efficient operations and use of resources.	5	4	3	2	1

Statement	Strongly Agree	Agree	Neither Agree Nor Disagree	Disagree	Strongly Disagree
7. The hospital administration works hard to increase the hospital's attractiveness to patients.	5	4	3	2	1
8. The hospital administration gets things done quickly.	5	4	3	2	1
9. The hospital serves all types of patients and patient problems.	5	4	3	2	1
10. The hospital serves as a source of health and human services for the entire community.	5	4	3	2	1

SECTION B

Statement	Strongly Agree	Agree	Neither Agree Nor Disagree	Disagree	Strongly Disagree
11. Hospital ambulatory care programs compete with physicians.	5	4	3	2	1
12. Hospital diagnostic services compete with physicians.	5	4	3	2	1
13. The hospital's involvement with prepaid plans (HMO's) is inappropriate.	5	4	3	2	1
14. The hospital's involvement with PPO's is inappropriate.	5	4	3	2	1
15. There is limited physician input in developing hospital policy.	5	4	3	2	1
16. There is inadequate attention paid to indigent care.	5	4	3	2	1

Statement	Strongly Agree	Agree	Neither Agree Nor Disagree	Disagree	Strongly Disagree
17. The efforts to recruit primary care physicians who can admit and refer patients to specialists are inadequate.	5	4	3	2	1
18. The hospital's goals are unclear or inconsistent.	5	4	3	2	1
19. The hospital's admissions policies are restrictive.	5	4	3	2	1
20. Physicians lack control over medical care decisions.	5	4	3	2	1

SECTION C

Statement	Strongly Agree	Agree	Neither Agree Nor Disagree	Disagree	Strongly Disagree
21. There are pressures to *not* use certain ancillary tests/ services.	5	4	3	2	1
22. The hospital exerts pressure to call in consulting physicians.	5	4	3	2	1
23. The hospital exerts pressure to make in-house referrals.	5	4	3	2	1
24. The hospital exerts pressure to discharge/transfer Medicare patients early.	5	4	3	2	1
25. The hospital exerts pressure to *not* admit indigent patients.	5	4	3	2	1
26. The hospital exerts pressure to transfer indigent patients to other hospitals.	5	4	3	2	1

Statement	Strongly Agree	Agree	Neither Agree Nor Disagree	Disagree	Strongly Disagree
27. The hospital restricts privileges or denies reappointment to "high cost" physicians.	5	4	3	2	1
28. The hospital is unwilling to form joint ventures with physicians.	5	4	3	2	1
29. The hospital fails to provide management assistance to physicians.	5	4	3	2	1
30. Hospital administration views physicians as "hospital labor."	5	4	3	2	1

SECTION D

31. Hospital administration fails to promote quality care.	5	4	3	2	1
32. Hospital administration fails to promote the hospital's image.	5	4	3	2	1
33. There are inadequate risk management efforts.	5	4	3	2	1
34. Inflexible rules hamper physician discretion in treating crisis cases.	5	4	3	2	1
35. There is uneven quality of hospital ancillary services (x-ray, lab, etc.)	5	4	3	2	1
36. There is unevern quality of hospital support services (housekeeping, dietary).	5	4	3	2	1

Statement	Strongly Agree	Agree	Neither Agree Nor Disagree	Disagree	Strongly Disagree
37. There is uneven quality of medical staff.	5	4	3	2	1
38. There is uneven quality of nursing staff.	5	4	3	2	1
39. There is an inadequate number of nurses to provide quality patient care.	5	4	3	2	1
40. The hospital fails to purchase equipment/technology requested.	5	4	3	2	1

SECTION E

Statement	Strongly Agree	Agree	Neither Agree Nor Disagree	Disagree	Strongly Disagree
41. The hospital fails to respond quickly to purchase requests.	5	4	3	2	1
42. There is inadequate maintenance of current equipment.	5	4	3	2	1
43. There is unavailability of beds.	5	4	3	2	1
44. There is unavailability of operating rooms.	5	4	3	2	1
45. The range of clinical services offered is inadequate.	5	4	3	2	1
46. The provision of patient education programs is inadequate.	5	4	3	2	1
47. The provision of community health programs is inadequate.	5	4	3	2	1
48. The provision of preventive health programs is inadequate.	5	4	3	2	1

Statement	Strongly Agree	Agree	Neither Agree Nor Disagree	Disagree	Strongly Disagree
49. The provision of services to the elderly is inadequate.	5	4	3	2	1
50. The quality assurance program is not as strong as it should be.	5	4	3	2	1

SECTION F

Statement	Strongly Agree	Agree	Neither Agree Nor Disagree	Disagree	Strongly Disagree
51. Hospital administration and physicians are in basic agreement on the overall goals of the institution.	5	4	3	2	1
52. The hospital views the physician as a competitor.	5	4	3	2	1
53. The hospital views the physician as a partner.	5	4	3	2	1
54. The hospital views the physician as an independent contractor.	5	4	3	2	1
55. The hospital views the physician as an employee.	5	4	3	2	1
56. The physician views the hospital as a "doctors' workshop."	5	4	3	2	1
57. Sufficient number of physicians are involved in hospital management and governance.	5	4	3	2	1
58. Physicians are sufficiently involved in the hospital's strategic planning process.	5	4	3	2	1
59. Physicians are called upon to provide input early in the decision-making process.	5	4	3	2	1

Statement	Strongly Agree	Agree	Neither Agree Nor Disagree	Disagree	Strongly Disagree
60. Physicians perceive the hospital's decision-making process to be fair.	5	4	3	2	1

SECTION G

Statement	Strongly Agree	Agree	Neither Agree Nor Disagree	Disagree	Strongly Disagree
61. The relative degree of power and influence among the hospital board, management and medical staff is appropriate.	5	4	3	2	1
62. Physician loyalty to the hospital is high.	5	4	3	2	1
63. The biggest threat to effective hospital-physician relationships are external economic and regulatory forces.	5	4	3	2	1
64. The biggest threat to effective hospital-physician relationships are internal disagreements among board, management and medical staff.	5	4	3	2	1
65. A key component of future success wil be joint hospital-physician organizations.	5	4	3	2	1
66. Our current medical staff organization structure is ineffective.	5	4	3	2	1
67. Our current mechanisms for managing conflict are ineffective.	5	4	3	2	1
68. The hospital uses its strategic plan to help guide everyday decision-making.	5	4	3	2	1

Statement	Strongly Agree	Agree	Neither Agree Nor Disagree	Disagree	Strongly Disagree
69. The physicians and hospital work together as a team.	5	4	3	2	1
70. The hospital enjoys strong physician leadership.	5	4	3	2	1

Please indicate your primary role within the hospital below:

_____ 1. Hospital executive/manager
_____ 2. Physician
_____ 3. Board member
_____ 4. Other (Please briefly indicate): _____

_____

THANK YOU.
PLEASE PLACE THE QUESTIONNAIRE IN THE ATTACHED
ENVELOPE MARKED "CONFIDENTIAL," AND GIVE IT TO THE
INTERVIEWER DURING YOUR INTERVIEW SESSION.

Results of Self-Administered Questionnaire

Table B.1 Summary of Hospital-Physician Questionnaire

Scale*	Average (Standard Deviation)	Range
Hospital responsiveness and support	3.6 (.64)	3.0–4.3
Leadership, teamwork, and decision making	3.5 (.62)	2.9–4.2
Admission policies	4.0 (.74)	3.3–4.8
Community health programs	3.8 (.63)	3.6–4.3
Lack of competition between hospital and physicians	3.8 (.62)	3.5–4.4
Hospital's treatment of physicians	3.7 (.61)	3.4–4.3
Physician recruitment	3.7 (.57)	3.2–4.2
Physician autonomy	4.0 (.63)	3.6–4.5
Appropriateness of managed care involvement	3.8 (.71)	2.5–4.3

Note: N = 130; 1 to 5 scale where 1 = low and 5 = high.
*Based on principal component analysis using varimax rotation. See following pages for further information on each scale and the individual items making up each scale.

Table B2. Further Statistical Information on Hospital-Physician Questionnaire

Factor	Eigen Value	Percent Variance	Cumulative Variance	Alpha's (Scale Reliability)
Hospital responsiveness and support	12.01	21.8	21.8	.87
Leadership, teamwork, and decision making	3.63	6.6	28.4	.84
Admission policies	2.99	5.4	33.9	.82
Community health programs	2.82	5.1	39.0	.77
Lack of competition between hospital and physicians	2.27	4.1	43.2	.78
Hospital's treatment of physicians	2.65	3.7	46.9	.78
Physician recruitment	1.99	3.6	50.5	.67
Physician autonomy	1.83	3.3	53.8	.71
Appropriateness of managed care involvement	1.56	2.8	56.7	.64

Table B.3 Items Making Up Each Scale

Hospital Responsiveness and Support

The hospital fails to respond quickly to purchase requests.*

There is inadequate maintenance of current equipment.

The hospital administration gets things done quickly.

The hospital fails to purchase equipment/technology requested.

There is uneven quality of hospital support services (housekeeping, dietary).

Physicians are sufficiently involved in the hospital's strategic planning process.

There is uneven quality of hospital ancillary services (x-ray, lab, etc.).

The quality assurance program is not as strong as it should be.

Physicians are called upon to provide input early in the decision-making process.

The hospital provides the needed equipment and services to support quality care.

Leadership, Teamwork, and Decision Making

The hospital enjoys strong physician leadership.

The biggest threat to effective hospital-physician relationships are internal disagreements among board, management, and medical staff.

The physicians and hospital work together as a team.

The biggest threat to effective hospital-physician relationships are external economic and regulatory forces.

The relative degree of power and influence among the hospital board, management, and medical staff is appropriate.

Our current medical staff organization structure is ineffective.

Sufficient numbers of physicians are involved in hospital management and governance.

Our current mechanisms for managing conflict are ineffective.

Physicians perceive the hospital's decision-making process to be fair.

Hospital administration and physicians are in basic agreement on the overall goals of the institution.

Admission Policies

The hospital exerts pressure to transfer indigent patients to other hospitals.

The hospital exerts pressure to not admit indigent patients.

There is inadequate attention paid to indigent care.

The hospital serves all types of patients and patient problems.

The hospital's admission policies are restrictive.

The hospital serves as a source of health and human services for the entire community.

Community Health Programs

The provision of community health programs is inadequate.

The provision of preventive health programs is inadequate.

Continued

Table B.3   Continued

The provision of patient education programs is inadequate.

The hospital uses its strategic plan to help guide everyday decision making.

Physicians lack control over medical care decisions.

Lack of Competition Between Hospital and Physicians

The hospital is careful not to compete with its medical staff.

Physician loyalty to the hospital is high.

The hospital provides the needed personnel to support quality care.

The hospital administration ensures cost-efficient operations and use of resources.

The hospital views the physician as a competitor.

The hospital provides the needed equipment and services to support quality care.

Hospital's Treatment of Physicians

There is an inadeqeuate number of nurses to provide quality patient care.

The hospital's goals are unclear or inconsistent.

Hospital administration views physicians as "hospital labor."

Sufficient numbers of physicians are involved in hospital management and governance.

There is unavailability of operating rooms.

Physician Recruitment

The efforts to recruit primary care physicians who can admit and refer patients to specialists are inadequate.

There are inadequate risk management efforts.

Our current medical staff organization structure is ineffective.

Hospital administration fails to promote quality care.

Physician Autonomy

The hospital exerts pressure to call in consulting physicians.

The hospital exerts pressure to make in-house referrals.

The hospital restricts privileges or denies reappointment to "high cost" physicians.

The hospital exerts pressure to discharge/transfer Medicare patients early.

Appropriateness of Managed Care Involvement

The hospital's involvement with prepaid plans (HMOs) is inappropriate.

The hospital's involvement with PPOs is inappropriate.

The hospital views the physician as an independent contractor.

The hospital is unwilling to form joint ventures with physicians.

*All negatively worded items were reverse scored.

APPENDIX C

Study Site Background
Narratives

CATHERINE MCAULEY HEALTH CENTER
(ST. JOSEPH MERCY HOSPITAL)

LOCATION: Ann Arbor, Michigan

OWNERSHIP: Not-for-profit religiously affiliated system member
              (Sisters of Mercy Health Corporation), medical
              school affiliated

SIZE: 554 beds (St. Joseph Mercy Hospital)

OCCUPANCY: 83 percent

KEY SERVICES: Broad range of services including cardiology,
              psychiatry, ambulatory care centers, adult and
              adolescent chemical dependency

Hospital Background and History

St. Joseph Mercy Hospital (Catherine McAuley Health Center) was
founded in 1911 by the Religious Sisters of Mercy at the request of local
University of Michigan physician department heads who needed a place
to treat their private patients. An Ann Arbor house was converted to
accommodate 11 beds. In 1924, Mercywood Hospital, a mental health
facility, was started. McAuley Health Center currently includes

1. 554-bed St. Joseph Mercy Hospital
2. the Reichert Health Building, which houses 120 physician offices and numerous outpatient services
3. Huron Oaks—a 40-bed residential chemical dependency facility
   for adults and adolescents
4. Alpha House—a 16-bed long-term care residential chemical dependency facility for adolescents
5. Mercywood Health Building—a 130-bed psychiatric hospital
6. several ambulatory care centers in the surrounding Brighton,
   Canton, and Plymouth communities

Overall, McAuley Health Center contains 740 beds in a state-of-the-art
facility.

An important aspect of McAuley's history and culture has been ongoing physician involvement. When the original hospital was started in 1911, physicians has offices in the building. As the hospital expanded, additional physician space was always included. This close physical proximity facilitated interaction between and among physicians, nurses, and executives.

McAuley Health Center is the largest member of the Mercy Health Services Corporation, a hospital and health care system headquartered in Farmington Hills, Michigan. The system owns 19 hospitals in Michigan, Iowa, and Indiana and has management contracts with an additional 7 hospitals. In addition, the system contains subsidiary corporations charged with providing care to the elderly and the development of managed care systems, among other things. McAuley Health Center is committed to the Sisters of Mercy Health Corporation's philosophy: "We dedicate our efforts to aid all persons in their striving for human wholeness—physically, psychologically, socially, and spiritually. We acknowledge that every person has the basic human right to needed health care."

Given the early influence of the University of Michigan physicians, McAuley Health Center serves as a major teaching and referral institution and currently has approximately 100 house staff.

Local Environment and Performance

Until recently, McAuley was relatively immune to major competitive forces due to its location as the only major community hospital and, therefore, the market leader in its area. In recent years, however, Henry Ford and other Detroit providers have considered expansion plans into the western suburbs of Detroit. In response, McAuley has seen the importance of extending their geographic domain. They also recognize the need to provide more cost-effective care, given the growing presence of HMOs and related managed care initiatives. Primarily a specialty-oriented hospital through the years, they now see the need to recruit additional primary care physicians in order to respond to the new practice environment.

Financially, McAuley continues to do well. Inpatient occupancy rates are holding in the area of 83 percent of staffed beds, and outpatient visits are growing at the rate of approximately 25 percent per year. The hospitals' operating margin, however, declined from 6.5 percent in 1985 to 2.3 percent in 1987, but rebounded to 5.5 percent in 1988. Its total net margin declined from 6.7 percent in 1985 to 2.8 percent in 1987, but increased to 6.3 percent in 1988.

Management Stability

McAuley has enjoyed good management stability: the current CEO has been at the institution 22 years (13 years as CEO), and the chief operating officer 8 years. The vice president for patient care has been in her position for 11 years, and most other senior-level and upper-level managers have been at McAuley for 7 to 8 years.

Medical Staff Organization and Physician Involvement

There are approximately 400 active staff members at McAuley, of whom 75 percent are board certified. Approximately 75 percent of the active members have appointments at other hospitals, but for the most part, McAuley is their primary hospital. The predominant form of practice in the community is solo practice (59 percent of the active staff); 24 percent are members of small two- or three-person partnerships. There is a part-time vice president for medical services, part-time section chiefs for the major clinical services, and a salaried full-time physician who serves as vice president of quality assurance.

The chief of the medical staff serves a two-year term, as does the vice chief of staff. Three physicians serve as board members of the hospital's 16-person governing board, and in addition, the chief of staff serves as a nonvoting member. The hospital CEO also serves as a voting member of the governing board. Several physicians also serve on the hospital's strategic planning committee. The president and board chair of the local independent practice association (IPA) attend board meetings as guests.

The Huron Valley Physicians' Association (HVPA) is a 450-member IPA. Of these physicians, 350 are on McAuley's staff, with the remaining on the staffs of surrounding area hospitals. The IPA has been in existence for approximately five years and serves as the business organization for the physicians. The IPA is the physician provider for a 78,000 member HMO, Care Choices.

Significant Accomplishments

Among the most frequently mentioned accomplishments involving hospital-physician relationships at McAuley in recent years are the following:

1. increasing patient care volume in the face of cutbacks in house staff hours. Medical staff members and management have worked harder and responded well.

2. the expansion of medical staff support for expanding the number of ambulatory sites, for recruiting primary care physicians

3. the completion of the Reichert physician office building

4. starting a sponsored primary care group practice to offer alternative practice opportunities to physicians. This was done with medical staff approval.

5. development of a new institutionwide focus on total quality management

Significant Problems and Challenges

Among the most frequently mentioned problems and challenges that McAuley has faced in recent years are the following:

1. integrating the hospital into the larger Sisters of Mercy Health Corporation system. Differences regarding ownership of the HMO represent one example of this challenge.

2. renegotiating exclusive contracts with hospital-based specialists. This has raised the generic issue of whether some physicians have been favored over others. The CEO's view is that these contracts are based on quality grounds and not economic criteria. Therefore, anytime that the medical staff does not want a contract renewed, the hospital is willing to negotiate contracts with new physicians.

3. developing alternative mechanisms for providing leadership in the various clinical departments. For example, should there be one head for all subgroups in a single department or subheads for individual departments within a larger division? The problem, in part, concerns the issue of small departments lacking consistent leadership from year to year. An ad hoc committee has been appointed to study the various options and recommend a solution.

4. facing the issue of more work for physicians given the existence of fewer residents

5. tensions between primary care physicians and subspecialists. There is a need for more primary care physicians, but some specialists have expressed some concern regarding this development.

6. the need to give more attention to the allocation of capital resources. Given that the medical center can no longer buy all equipment and technology, they are asking physicians to assist in raising additional funds for desired equipment.

Keys to the Future

Looking ahead to the next couple of years, McAuley believes that the following decisions and events will prove critical:

1. the need to clarify the role that the Huron Valley Physicians' Association will play in the future evolution of health care in the Ann Arbor area. Options include remaining in their current IPA structure, becoming a multispecialty group practice, or assuming some other organizational form.

2. the undertaking of a project designed to envision and implement the desired medical practice environment for McAuley in the Ann Arbor area in the year 2000. This project, called PHYSICIANS 2000, is jointly sponsored by the Health Center, the Huron Valley Physicians' Association, and the hospital medical staff. Eight priority areas have already been identified: quality of care; the clinical practice environment; the economics of medical practice; quality of life, the malpractice situation; relationships among physicians, other health care professionals, and managers; influence processes (such as with the state legislators); and the relationship with the University of Michigan Medical Center.

3. the need to continue to aggressively build volume in order to support the medical center campus and preclude additional competition from coming into the area. As part of this, the hospital has instituted physician liaison groups who are interviewing physician office managers to determine how the medical center can best meet the needs of McAuley physicians.

4. issues related to the relative roles to be played in regard to indigent care and provision of services to the elderly.

CROUSE-IRVING MEMORIAL HOSPITAL

LOCATION: Syracuse, New York

OWNERSHIP: Not-for-profit independent, medical school affiliated

SIZE: 612 beds

OCCUPANCY: 93 percent

KEY SERVICES: Broad range of services including cardiology,
                         obstetrics, outpatient surgery

Hospital Background and History

Crouse-Irving Memorial has a long history of service to the Syracuse community dating back to the late 1800s when it was founded as a women's and children's hospital. A key event in its history was the merger of Crouse-Irving Hospital and Syracuse Memorial Hospital in 1968. The medical staff leadership of both institutions played a key role in the merger, which was heavily supported by the community.

Crouse-Irving Memorial is largely a specialty-oriented institution but with a strong internal medicine component. It has distinct strengths in cardiology, obstetrics, and outpatient surgery. It has recently initiated a strategic planning process designed to better position itself for the future, including the need to expand into the northern section of its service area.

The hospital has recently completed a $37 million building project adding two medical-surgical floors. Crouse-Irving Memorial also operates two one-day surgery centers, an adolescent substance-abuse treatment program, a physician referral service, three affiliated family health care centers, an off-site adult and adolescent chemical dependency center, and a home care agency offering both durable medical equipment and in-home personal health services. Due to a critical shortage of qualified nurses, the hospital has closed 55 beds, including 36 of the newly constructed beds. To help address the nurse shortage problem, the hospital has developed a "Tuition's on us" program whereby qualified students are granted a tuition-free education in exchange for a commitment to work at Crouse-Irving Memorial for three years after graduation.

Local Environment and Performance

The Syracuse environment can best be described as being ten years ahead of the country in regard to the degree of regulation, and ten years behind the country in regard to the degree of competition. New York, one of the most regulated states in the country, presents major challenges for Crouse-Irving Memorial—100 percent of their inpatient revenue is controlled by the state through a new all-payer, all-patient diagnose-related group (DRG) system implemented in 1988. Recent legislation cutting back on the number of hours to be worked by residents coupled with the shortage of nurses poses additional staffing challenges that will have to be addressed, at least in part, by greater work effort by current attending physicians. The state has also initiated a system whereby each hospital must report its critical incidents to the State Department of Health, which in turn refers such information to each hospital board member. The net result is that the hospital is frequently placed in the position of implementing state regulations, resulting in increased tension between the hospital and its physicians.

There is relatively little direct competition in the Syracuse area. This is in part due to stringent health planning legislation throughout the 1970s, which resulted in a reduction of the number of hospitals in the area from seven to four, plus the continuance of a Veterans Administration hospital. At present, there is relatively little HMO or managed care activity. Reflecting the lack of a competitive environment, the executives of the four hospitals meet monthly as the hospital executive council to discuss mutual plans and opportunities and how they might best coordinate services in the area. In similar fashion, the medical directors of the hospitals meet under the auspices of the hospital executive council to coordinate recredentialing and other medical staff activities jointly.

The hospital has operated at an approximately 93 percent occupancy for the past several years and broke even financially in 1987. Given the reimbursement and regulatory environment in the state, however, the hospital lost $6.7 million in 1988, representing about 3 percent of the hospital's total net margin.

Management Stability

Crouse-Irving Memorial has enjoyed considerable management stability. The chief executive officer has been at the hospital for 25 years, the last 9 as CEO. The president of the hospital board has served for 15 years. The medical director has been associated with the hospital for over 20 years, as have many of the other medical staff leaders.

Medical Staff Organization and Physician Involvement

Crouse-Irving Memorial has 500 active staff members, of whom 94 percent are board certified and 90 percent have appointments at one or more other hospitals. Approximately 56 percent of the physicians' practices are solo; an additional 27 percent are members of two- or three-person partnerships. The hospital has a full-time paid vice president for medical affairs, who also serves as head of the medical care evaluation (i.e., quality assurance) committee. Part-time paid chiefs, appointed by the board, exist for all of the major clinical areas. The president and president elect of the medical staff serve two-year terms of office. There is no direct hospital HMO or PPO (preferred provider organization) sponsorship, and there are currently no economic joint ventures between the hospital and its physicians, although a few are under consideration.

There are three physicians on the hospital's 26-person governing board, of whom one is a voting member. The hospital CEO is a nonvoting member of the board. There is a relatively inactive strategic planning committee, which also has the participation of three physicians. Hospital board members regularly attend meetings of the medical staff credentials committee, executive committee, and quality assurance committee. There is no parallel organization of the medical staff such as an IPA, PPA, or joint physician-hospital organization.

Significant Accomplishments

Among the significant accomplishments associated with the hospital-physician relationship in recent years at Crouse-Irving Memorial are the following:

1. the integration of the quality assurance functions of the medical staff with the quality assurance functions of the hospital's clinical support services

2. an affiliation with several urgent care centers in the east and north of the service area despite some physician opposition

3. the creation of a joint hospital-physician marketing committee, which has served to improve relationships with physicians

4. the ability to integrate five specialty offices into a single ambulatory medical center in order to increase the hospital's referral base

5. improved communication with physicians in which hospital administration has admitted its mistakes. The openness and candor exhibited by hospital administration has enabled it to

maintain relatively good relationships with its physicians despite the difficulties posed by operating in a highly regulated environment.

Significant Problems and Challenges

Among the most frequently mentioned problems and challenges faced by Crouse-Irving Memorial are the following:

1. the reimbursement and budgetary pressures exerted by the highly intense regulatory environment of New York State
2. a recent suit initiated by a anesthesiologist whose privileges were restricted by the hospital. The findings of the medical staff executive committee were supported by the board, and overall the review process served the hospital well
3. the acute shortage of nurses
4. an association with the urgent care centers in the north end of the county that raised problems with some physicians who perceived it as a competitive threat
5. dealing with some malpractice issues involving some orthopedic surgeons

Keys to the Future

Looking ahead to the next couple of years, Crouse-Irving Memorial believes that the following issues will be pivotal in determining the future evolution of hospital-physician relationships:

1. The continuing reimbursement pressures will cause the hospital to rethink its fee-for-service contracts with its hospital-based specialists (i.e., the radiologists, pathologists, and anesthesiologists).
2. The reimbursement and other economic controls will make it difficult for hospital administration to continue to implement its philosophy of providing all medical staff members with equal access resources.
3. The hospital will need to deal with the cutbacks in residency hours—perhaps by hiring some nurse practitioners.
4. The hospital will need to deal with competitive pressures developing between cardiology groups on the hospital staff.
5. Some key people believe that the relationship between the hospital and its physicians could get worse over the next year or two given the pressures cited above. At the very least, the relationship will be strongly tested.

LEONARD MORSE HOSPITAL

LOCATION: Natick, Massachusetts

OWNERSHIP: Not-for-profit independent district (city)

SIZE: 259 beds

OCCUPANCY: 67 percent

KEY SERVICES: Basic medical-surgical, adult and child psychiatry, respiratory, home health

---

Hospital Background and History

Leonard Morse is located in Natick, Massachusetts, a community of about 35,000 about 16 miles west of Boston. The hospital was founded in the late 1800s with funds left from the will of a local community leader. The hospital has a tradition of providing friendly community-oriented services with physicians who are well established in the community. The hospital offers the usual range of services, including an adult and child psychiatry program and an alcohol and substance abuse program.

Leonard Morse is a private 501(C)3 hospital with a unique requirement under the will that seven trustees be elected from the town of Natick. The hospital has had a relatively weak politically oriented board, which, coupled with CEO turnover, has resulted in physicians having more unchecked influence than usual. At the same time, physicians believe they have had to exert such influence due to the infighting among the trustees and the instability caused by CEO turnover. The board has enjoyed stronger leadership in the past few years and has supported the most recent CEO in a joint effort to develop more effective relationships with physicians, in particular with regard to managed care issues.

Local Environment and Performance

Surrounded by seven hospitals in the western suburbs of Boston, Leonard Morse operates in a highly competitive environment. Several of the competing hospitals have residency programs with Boston teaching hospitals. The competing hospitals are generally somewhat larger and somewhat more specialized than Leonard Morse, offering such services as cardiac catherization and radiation therapy.

Leonard Morse has been slower than its competition in getting involved with managed care because of medical staff opposition. Approximately eight years ago, the hospital, in conjunction with three other hospitals, developed Family Health Plan, a local HMO. The plan paid the hospitals based on charges, and physicians on discounted fees. One hospital raised its charges to the point that it began to bankrupt the HMO. The plan was on the verge of bankruptcy and was taken over by a larger, more successful HMO—the Pilgrim Health Plan. Leonard Morse physicians were extremely upset with this development because they felt that the hospitals got most of the money from the venture, while the physicians' fees were inadequate. They felt that the hospital should not have supported the transfer to Pilgrim Health Plan. The hospital felt it had to stay involved for competitive purposes. The hospital also enjoyed some support from its primary care physicians who saw the need for developing larger panels of patients. The board supported administration in its stance. There remains some lingering suspicion and lack of trust on the part of some physicians toward the hospital as a result of this experience.

Leonard Morse also operates in the highly regulated environment of Massachusetts. It often takes several years to clear the review hurdles for new programs and services. For example, it has taken the hospital several years to negotiate payment rates for a child development center. Most recently, hospitals in this state are being paid for volume increases, which in turn has stimulated more competition for patients and physicians.

The hospital's occupancy has been averaging 65 percent over the past four years, declining from 72 percent in 1985 to 61 percent in 1988. Inpatient admissions have declined somewhat, as have visits to the hospital's emergency room. In a state where 60–70 percent of the hospitals are losing money, Leonard Morse Hospital has made a small profit from operations and done somewhat better when nonoperating income is added in.

Management Stability

There has been considerable CEO turnover at Leonard Morse over the years, with CEO tenure averaging about five years. The current CEO has been in her position for four years. A new chief operating officer has been on board for approximately two years. A new vice president for nursing has just been appointed.

Medical Staff Organization and Physician Involvement

Leonard Morse has 95 active staff physicians, of whom 82 percent are board certified. It has a reasonable balance of specialists and primary care physicians. Of the active staff physicians, 90 percent practice as solo practitioners or in two- or three-person partnerships. Approximately 80 percent have appointments at two or more hospitals, but approximately 70 percent of these are primarily loyal to, and admit a majority of their patients to, Leonard Morse.

The hospital does not have a vice president for medical affairs or a medical director, nor does the hospital have any full-time or part-time paid section chiefs. There is an IPA established to oversee an HMO contract with the Tufts Associated Health Plan. The hospital also has a fully capitated contract with Pilgrim HMO for a panel of 5,000 members. The hospital had established a joint venture corporation with its physicians for the purpose of joint planning. A respiratory home health care program was initiated. More recently, the physicians and hospital have incorporated a physician-hospital organization for the specific purpose of contracting and managing HMO contracts together. The medical staff president and president elect each serve two-year terms. Of the seven elected town board members, one is a physician who practices at Leonard Morse. In addition, five physicians are involved as members of the board's strategic planning committee. The hospital CEO cannot be a member of the governing board because of the will. She does participate as an observer at the medical staff executive committee meeting, and she also attends the patient care review committee meetings. The chief operating officer attends the credentials, quality assurance, and utilization review committees of the medical staff.

Significant Accomplishments

The most frequently mentioned accomplishments involving the relationship between the hospital and its physicians in the past couple of years are the following:

1. working through physician opposition to the hospital's involvement in Pilgrim Health Plan. In the long run, several hospital observers believe it will help bind the physicians closer to the hospital. They believe the hospital and physicians will emerge stronger as a result of having gone through the experience.
2. the establishment of a number of successful joint ventures between the hospital and its physician corporation (Allied Enterprises and Medical Services). Joint ventures have been launched

in the areas of respiratory home health and development of a primary care practice. With the new PHO in place, plans are to jointly contract with and manage HMO contracts.

3. maintaining a generally positive public image in the community during some rather difficult times

4. some success in recruiting additional primary care physicians

5. successfully recruiting three new obstetricians, building a new labor, delivery, recovery postpartum (LDRP—single room maternity) unit, and further developing its psychiatry and alcohol services to help attract HMO patients

Significant Problems and Challenges

The most frequently mentioned challenges and problems faced by the hospital in the most recent year or two are the following:

1. the acute shortage of nurses and the changes in nursing practice. As a result, the hospital has relied more on LPNs and aides.

2. the physician opposition to the hospital's participation in the Pilgrim Health Plan. There remains a residue of mistrust and suspicion due to physician beliefs that the hospital did well under the previous plan at physicians' expense.

3. maintaining fiscal solvency in the increasingly competitive and regulatory environment that the hospital faces

4. dealing with higher malpractice coverage limits

5. difficulty in recruiting new physicians in a number of areas, including pediatrics and cardiology, due to fear of competition from existing specialists

6. the need for stronger medical staff leadership and continued board development

Keys to the Future

In looking ahead to the next year or so, respondents felt the following events would be critical to the evolving hospital-physician relationship at Leonard Morse:

1. New medical staff structures in which hospital-physician incentives are economically aligned must be developed. In this regard, the future of the physician-hospital corporation is critical. The hospital committed $100,000 towards the development of

this physician-hospital organization to contract with and manage alternative delivery system contracts, and it is expected that this structure will be the mechanism by which the hospital and its physicians can successfully compete in the managed care market.

2. Some believe that it may be possible to develop a group practice as a subsidiary corporation under AEMS. This is seen as providing a better structure for competing in the managed care environment.

3. In general, how well the hospital and its medical staff deal with managed care issues and the associated physician recruitment issues are seen as keys to its success.

LEXINGTON MEDICAL CENTER

LOCATION: West Columbia, South Carolina

OWNERSHIP: Not-for-profit independent district

SIZE: 292 beds

OCCUPANCY: 75 percent

KEY SERVICES: General medical-surgical, strong primary care base

---

Hospital Background and History

Lexington Medical Center recently changed its name from Lexington County Hospital to Lexington Medical Center in order to communicate a more positive image and to reflect a relatively broad range of services offered. Founded in 1970, the hospital has a reputation as a progressive, innovative community hospital with a strong primary care base. Lexington also operates a day hospital, a 391-bed nursing home, and a retirement community.

A key event in the hospital's history was the relatively recent replacement of the former CEO. This individual, who led the hospital's growth in its early years, was perceived as trying to do too much himself, not sufficiently involving the medical staff in decision making, and becoming overly involved in diversification activities that lost money. A new CEO has opened doors of communication and has begun to reestablish trust and respect between the hospital and the physicians. This has been facilitated by the adoption of a strong, formal strategic planning process with significant physician involvement.

Local Environment and Performance

Lexington is one of four hospitals in a rapidly growing area of approximately 450,000. At this point, the competition is not intense but may be growing. There is some HMO competition developing. Lexington is generally not seen as the preferred hospital because of an early unwillingness to discount services and a perception on the part of some employers that the hospital is not as full service as others.

Inpatient occupancy has averaged approximately 78 percent over the past three years but has declined from 81.8 percent in 1985 to 74.8

percent in 1987. Admissions declined from 13,800 to 12,485. Outpatient visits have held steady at approximately 26,000. Lexington's operating margins over the three years have been 6.4, 1.4, and 2.4 percent, and its total net margins have been 7.9, 3, and 3.6 percent.

Management Stability

The original CEO was with the hospital for approximately twenty years. He was succeeded by his assistant, who had been with the hospital for about one year and has now served as CEO for about a year and a half. The vice president for nursing has been at the hospital for a total of a year and a half. The board chairman has been a member of the board for five years and has served as chair for the past two years. Most of the physician leaders have been with the staff for approximately eight to ten years.

Medical Staff Organization and Physician Involvement

Lexington has an active staff of 166 physicians, 82 percent of whom are board certified and 80 percent of whom have appointments at one or more other hospitals in the area. A core group of about 75 physicians, however, primarily use Lexington. Of the active staff, 86 percent practice in solo settings or in small partnerships and groups of not more than five physicians. There is no full-time medical director or executive vice president for medical affairs, although there is a part-time paid medical director for quality assurance. There are no full-time or part-time paid section chiefs. The hospital does not have an IPA or physician-hospital organization but is involved in selected joint ventures with its physicians.

The president of the medical staff serves a two-year term. Three physicians serve as voting members of the hospital's 21-member board including the chief of staff. Governing board members attend quality assurance and utilization review committee meetings of the medical staff. The CEO is not a member of the board but does serve as an observer at the medical executive committee and regularly attends the quality assurance committee of the medical staff. The physicians were instrumental in encouraging the hospital to form a strategic planning committee and are actively involved in the process; five members of the committee are physicians, five are from the administration, and five from the board. This process is further facilitated by retreats held twice a year.

Significant Accomplishments

Among the most frequently mentioned significant accomplishments growing out of the hospital-physician relationship at Lexington are the following:

1. adoption of an active formal strategic planning process. This process has already led to plans for development of new services such as a cath lab and linear accelerator.
2. successful resolution of a quality assurance problem involving the limitation of a doctor's privileges for inappropriate use of antibiotics
3. the current support given to the new CEO as he attempts to open up communication and move the hospital forward
4. the shift in the hospital's strategy to avoid competing with its physicians on diversification efforts and instead work to support existing physicians
5. the decision to sign for their first HMO contract

Significant Problems and Challenges

Among the most frequently reported challenges and problems facing the hospital-physician relationship over the past year or two are the following:

1. the problems associated with the removal of the previous CEO
2. the hospital's diversification efforts into the day hospital and the retirement center, which has resulted in a $2.5 million loss
3. the shortage of nurses and technicians
4. reorganization of the nursing staff, which was opposed by some physicians
5. resolution of the antibiotic privileges issue, which involved the board and joint conference committee

Keys to the Future

Among the future events that are seen as affecting hospital-physician relationships at Lexington are the following:

1. working with physicians on joint venture possibilities to avoid the physicians starting on their own such new initiatives as ambulatory surgery and a birthing center

2. the need to attract some additional physicians
3. negotiating contracts for exclusive services
4. dealing with the increasing managed care environment
5. a general sense that the relationships will get stronger given the active strategic planning process that has been initiated

NORTH MONROE HOSPITAL

LOCATION: Monroe, Louisiana

OWNERSHIP: Investor-owned (Hospital Corporation of America)

SIZE: 190 beds

OCCUPANCY: 75 percent

KEY SERVICES: General medical-surgical, cardiac catherization, laser surgery, women and children's pavilion, adolescent psychiatry

---

Hospital Background and History

Monroe is a community of approximately 120,000 people with a larger attachment area of approximately 358,000 people in northeast Louisiana. The initiative for the hospital came from a group of physicians who were dissatisfied with the other major hospital in the community. They approached Hospital Corporation of America (HCA), who agreed to build a new facility in the growing north end of town in 1983. In 1984 a multispecialty clinic representing approximately 18 physicians moved from the competing hospital to North Monroe. This switch played a significant role in establishing North Monroe's credibility and in helping to steadily increase its market share. The clinic served as a catalyst for recruiting other high-quality physicians to the staff.

North Monroe is a community hospital with growing tertiary care capabilities. For a small community hospital it is unusual in the breadth and depth of its services. For example, it offers cardiac catherization, MRI, and laser surgery and has plans for open heart surgery. It also has a medical research department in which physicians conduct clinical drug studies. North Monroe physicians have also made breakthroughs in the treatment of lung cancer and have trained doctors from around the country in this new technique. The hospital places a great deal of emphasis on patient service and on projecting a high-quality image in the community.

Local Environment and Performance

There is considerable competition between North Monroe and a neighboring 400-bed long-established Catholic hospital. In addition, the

Monroe area has a 200-bed community hospital, a 225-bed state charity hospital, and a 90-bed psychiatric hospital.

The initial polarization caused by physicians splitting off from the Catholic hospital was intensified by the subsequent move of the multi-specialty clinic physicians. These two hospitals continue to compete for physicians and patients through new service and facility development. North Monroe has bought several million dollars of new equipment to upgrade facilities and technologies to meet emerging physician needs.

As a result of the above, the hospital has steadily increased its occupancy over the past five years, from a low of around 30 percent in 1984 to 75 percent in 1988. In 1988 its operating margin was 7.0 percent, and its total net margin 3.8 percent. These figures were down somewhat from 8.7 and 7.5 percent, respectively, in 1985. From 1985 to 1988 inpatient admissions grew significantly, from approximately 1,000 in 1985 to over 5,000 in 1988. Outpatient visits doubled from 6,600 to approximately 13,500.

Management Stability

North Monroe has experienced considerable management turnover, it has gone through four CEOs since its opening in 1983. At the time of the research the incumbent CEO, who had helped to nurture strong physician relationships and guide the hospital's growth, was in the process of leaving to take a significant career advancement opportunity with another system. This CEO, however, had been at the hospital for four years and during that period had exerted a major influence on physician relationships and on the hospital's growth.

Medical Staff Organization and Physician Involvement

The hospital has an active medical staff of 93 physicians, of whom 63 percent are board certified. It is a young staff, with many physicians in their late 30s and early 40s. While approximately 100 percent of the active staff practice at one or more other community hospitals, about one-third of these are primarily loyal to North Monroe. About 35 percent of the physicians are solo practitioners; another 30 percent are in two- or three-person partnerships; 7 percent are members of small four- or five-person groups; 20 percent are members of six- to fifteen-physician groups; and 8 percent are members of groups of physicians having sixteen or more members.

The hospital does not have a medical director or vice president for medical affairs or any paid full-time or part-time clinical chiefs. The president of the staff and president elect currently serve one-year terms. There are no hospital-sponsored HMOs or PPOs and relatively little joint venture activity with the exception of a breast clinic. There is no parallel organization such as an independent practice association or professional practice association. Five physicians serve as voting members of the hospital's eleven-member governing board. The terms of office are for five years. Over 40 physicians and community leaders were involved in the hospital's initial strategic planning effort in 1985, and physicians continue to be involved in strategic planning activities. The hospital CEO also serves as a voting member of the governing board and regularly attends meetings of the medical staff's credentials committee, quality assurance committee, and utilization review committee.

Significant Accomplishments

Among the most frequently mentioned accomplishments associated with hospital-physician relationships at North Monroe in the past couple of years are the following:

1. successful recruitment of seven new physicians and a highly regarded nuclear medicine specialist
2. the approval of an open heart surgery program
3. significant strides made in becoming a regional medical center
4. construction of a new 30-bed women and children's unit and a 48-bed additional adolescent psychiatric pavilion
5. effectively dealing with some difficult issues of physician credentialing

Significant Problems and Challenges

Among the most frequently mentioned problems and challenges faced by North Monroe are the following:

1. conflict and litigation involving a medical staff member regarding purchase of land for an additional office
2. a shortage of nurses and inadequate training
3. credentialing issues, such as what ENTs can do versus general surgeons
4. the need for continued acceptance of the institution on the part of the community
5. the recent replacement of the highly regarded CEO

Keys to the Future

Looking ahead to the next couple of years, North Monroe believes that the following issues will be central to determining the future evolution of hospital-physician relationships:

1. Physicians must be assisted in meeting their economic needs. This will probably involve more joint venture activity. If successful, the hospital feels it can be the leading major medical center in the northeast Louisiana area by 1991.

2. In order to accomplish the above, it may be necessary to devote more resources and attention to physicians who are not a part of the primary clinic on the hospital's campus. This may cause some friction with the clinic physicians but will be supported by the nonclinic physicians.

3. A better job needs to be done in grooming younger physicians for staff involvement and leadership.

4. Continued emphasis needs to be given to recruiting new physicians in selected areas such as vascular surgery.

5. Continued attention needs to be given to involving the physicians in decision making and encouraging them to make more of the decisions they should be making.

6. It is important that a physician-sensitive administrator be recruited to continue to guide the institution.

PROVIDENCE MEDICAL CENTER

LOCATION: Seattle, Washington

OWNERSHIP: Not-for-profit religiously affiliated system member (Sisters of Providence Health Corporation)

SIZE: 376 beds

OCCUPANCY: 68 percent

KEY SERVICES: Broad range of services including cardiology, cardiovascular surgery heart institute, psychiatry, primary care clinic network, home health and hospice.

Hospital Background and History

Providence Medical Center is one of seventeen not-for-profit institutions owned by Sisters of Providence Health Corporation. The hospital was the first in Seattle, founded in 1877 as a cottage hospital serving the pioneer community in the downtown area. Over the years, Providence has grown into a referral center for a number of specialties, including cardiology, cardiovascular surgery, respiratory care, rehabilitation medicine, and psychiatry. The hospital offers a wide range of services, from the Providence Heart Institute, to a network of primary care clinics, home health care, occupational medicine, and hospice programs. Providence reflects the Church's gospel values to serve all those in need. As a result, it is a major provider of care to the poor and medically indigent in the Seattle area.

Local Environment and Performance

Operating in a rate review state, combined with strong competition from at least three or four other teaching affiliated hospitals and serving a high percentage of Medicaid and Medicare patients (approximately 60 percent), has placed financial strains on the institution. Approximately 80 percent of their payments are not tied to their costs. As a result, the hospital recently initiated a $3 million overhead cutback including a reduction of middle-level and upper-level management staff. The Sisters of Providence System, overall, is facing the same pressures and recognizes the need for possible trade-offs regarding such alternatives as renovating older facilities, developing new services, and supporting the financial needs of weaker facilities.

Despite the financial, regulatory, and competitive pressures noted above, Providence has maintained its occupancy at around 68 percent over the past four years. Its operating margins, while declining, remain positive. For example, between 1985 and 1988, the hospital's operating margin declined from 5.4 to 0.2 percent, and its total net margin declined from 5.5 percent in 1985 to 0.15 percent in 1988. Inpatient admissions have grown from 13,228 in 1985 to 16,924 in 1988. Outpatient visits more than doubled between 1985 and 1988.

Management Stability

The hospital has enjoyed reasonable management stability over the past decade. The current CEO has been in the position for 9 years, the vice president for nursing approximately 8 years, the senior associate for 6 years, and the CFO for 12 years. The director of medical education has been associated with the hospital for approximately 12 years, and many of the medical staff leaders and section chiefs have been associated with the hospital from 18 to 20 years. A new vice president for medical affairs/ medical director was hired in the past year.

Medical Staff Organization and Physician Involvement

Providence has 324 active staff physicians, of whom 77 percent are board certified and 80 percent have appointments at one or more other hospitals. Many of these physicians admit patients to a major competing hospital as well as to Providence. Approximately 45 percent of the active staff physicians practice in groups of 16 or more physicians, and an additional 20 percent are in smaller groups. Part of the relatively high percentage of doctors practicing in groups is accounted for by a 50-physician multispecialty group practice (Pacmed), which recently affiliated with the hospital.

The hospital has a full-time paid vice president for medical affairs/ medical director and a full-time director of medical education. None of the section chiefs, however, are salaried, although there are a few part-time salaried department heads in such areas as cardiology, respiratory care, and critical care. The medical staff president and president elect serve one-year terms.

Physicians serve on the hospital's foundation board, which serves as both a fund-raising and advisory board. The Providence System has a centralized governance structure of eight individuals composed mainly of sisters. There are no physicians on the corporate board. Physicians were very actively involved in a comprehensive strategic planning initiative several years ago. This involved 15 physicians and 5 managers. The CEO attends medical staff executive committee meetings as an ex officio member but does not regularly attend credentials, quality assurance, or utilization review committee meetings.

The hospital is involved in both HMO and PPO sponsorship in association with four other Catholic systems in Washington State. The Sisters of Providence have a taxable organization that Providence has used for several joint ventures with its physicians, including an office building and MRI.

Significant Accomplishments

The most frequently mentioned accomplishments growing out of the hospital-physician relationship at Providence in recent years are the following:

1. expansion of the heart center and cardiovascular services, providing increased services and improved access
2. successful development of the primary care clinic network. This network has served as an important source of referrals for the institution.
3. renovation and general improvement of the hospital's physical plant
4. the willingness of the CEO to share problems and issues with the medical staff executive committee. The hospital is developing a team effort to deal with the challenges that they face.
5. improvements in the hospital's quality assurance program, including use of a software methodology to facilitate quality review

Significant Problems and Challenges

The most frequently mentioned challenges and opportunities that the hospital faced include the following:

1. improving the relationship between physicians and nurses, particularly in regard to charting and interpersonal relationships between nurses and physicians. The problem has been further complicated by the shortage of nurses.
2. working to incorporate the 50-member Pacmed group into the hospital's operating structure and philosophy. The Pacmed

group usually practices with residents providing much of the care—different from the prevailing pattern of practice in the hospital.

3. dealing with the growing financial pressures exerted by regulatory, competitive, and managed care forces

4. overcoming the hospital's image problem of primarily serving poor patients and, therefore, losing regular paying patients to competing hospitals

5. reducing the amount of time to make decisions

Keys to the Future

Among the items more frequently mentioned as being critical to the future evolution of hospital-physician relationships at Providence are the following:

1. determining how the hospital and physicians can work together given the growing financial pressures faced by both groups. Some tough choices will have to be made. Some people believe it is likely to get worse before the relationship gets better, with the possibility of some splits developing among the staff.

2. working to improve relationships between physicians and nurses

3. working to better integrate the 50-member Pacmed group physicians into the hospital

SCRIPPS MEMORIAL HOSPITAL

LOCATION: La Jolla, California

OWNERSHIP: Not-for-profit system member (Scripps Memorial Hospitals)

SIZE: 476 beds

OCCUPANCY: 70 percent

KEY SERVICES: Broad range of services including a cardiovascular institute, trauma center, eye institute, chemical dependency center, cancer center

Hospital Background and History

Scripps Memorial Hospital is located in La Jolla, California about ten miles from downtown San Diego. It is the largest hospital in a three-hospital system formed as a result of a corporate restructuring seven years ago. Scripps enjoys a reputation as a high-quality institution with a highly skilled medical staff. A turning point in its evolution occurred in 1976 when, upon the recommendation of a consultant, the hospital reduced its board size from 30 to 8 and hired a new CEO. The goal was to build a more business-oriented hospital and, at the same time, be responsive to physician needs. Physicians were influential in making these changes, having felt that their input into decision making was previously lacking. The hospital presently offers a variety of tertiary, secondary, and primary care services, including a cardiovascular institute (open heart surgery, two cath labs), a trauma center, Mericos Eye Institute, McDonald Center (a chemical dependency treatment center), and Stevens Cancer Center.

Local Environment and Performance

Scripps operates in a highly competitive environment surrounded by three or four major competing hospitals. A university hospital satellite is scheduled to be built within two blocks of Scripps over the coming two years. There is also considerable pressure on physician incomes given the high numbers of physicians in the area and the growth in managed care. The hospital is currently involved in approximately 40 HMO/PPO contracts, which comprise about 25 percent of their business. The hospital must also contend with state MediCal payment limits.

Scripps has done well to date operating in the competitive environment. Over the past four years, occupancy has averaged 69 percent. The hospital's operating margins for 1985, 1986, 1987, and 1988 were 7.5, 6.8, 7.2, and 7.2 percent, respectively. Its total net margins for 1986, 1987, and 1988 were 5.3, 5.2, and 4.8 percent, respectively. Inpatient admissions have increased slightly, while outpatient visits have grown by 50 percent.

Management Stability

The hospital has enjoyed considerable management stability. The CEO of the holding company has been with Scripps for 12 years, and the CEO of Scripps Memorial Hospital has been in his position for 10 years. In addition, the chief operating officer of the hospital has been present for 10 years. Most physician leaders have been affiliated with the institution for 15 to 20 years.

Medical Staff Organization and Physician Involvement

There are 740 physicians on the staff at Scripps, of whom 80 percent have appointments at two or more hospitals. Three hundred practice primarily at Scripps, and 90 percent of these are board certified. Fifty percent of the physicians practice as solo practitioners or in groups of two or three.

The chief of staff (president), chief of staff elect, and department heads are elected for two-year terms. All receive some stipend from medical staff dues. There are no hospital-employed physician administrators. The eight-member hospital board of trustees includes one physician, chosen by the board, with informal medical staff and administration input. A board member attends the monthly executive medical committee, and the hospital COO attends selected medical staff committee meetings.

XIMED is the physicians' corporation, established in 1979 so that physicians could carry out economic activities collectively. Its 250 members account for 85 percent of the admissions to Scripps, and membership is available only to physicians who use Scripps as their primary hospital. Physicians pay annual dues for a CEO, part-time medical director, and staff. XIMED does provider contracting, joint ventures with the hospital, group purchasing, etc.

Presently, neither Scripps nor XIMED sponsors an HMO or PPO, but both contract independently and a joint program is under discussion. Their joint ventures include a 215,000 square foot medical office building, an executive health and fitness program, and a sports medicine program. The hospital and XIMED have formed a joint corporation (50-50 ownership split), Scripps Memorial Healthcare.

Significant Accomplishments

The most frequently mentioned significant accomplishments associated with the hospital-physician relationships at Scripps during the past year or two are the following:

1. successful development of the medical office building through joint cooperation between XIMED and the hospital
2. development of XIMED itself to deal with economic issues facing physicians and the hospital
3. upgrading the hospital's quality assurance activities
4. development of successful joint ventures such as the fitness and sports center
5. the continued financial success of the hospital given the competitive and turbulent environment

Significant Problems and Challenges

The following are the most frequently reported significant challenges and problems that Scripps and its physicians are dealing with:

1. the lack of staffing in certain areas of the hospital such as ICU nurses and staffing in radiology. At the same time, staffing may need to be further cut in some areas due to the economic pressures.
2. the ability to allocate resources in the future to meet growing needs and demands
3. concern that meeting the expansion needs of the two satellite hospitals may deplete needed resources at Scripps Memorial
4. initial problems in getting the hospital to recognize XIMED
5. improving the surgery scheduling system. A task force is currently working on this problem.

Keys to the Future

Among the most important items mentioned regarding the future evolution of hospital-physician relationships at Scripps are the following:

1. Due to the economic and competitive environment, many observers felt the relationship will be challenged in the coming year or two. In order to maintain the effectiveness of the relationship, it will be necessary to do more joint activities. The XIMED-hospital relationship is seen as crucial here along with the ability to develop successful joint ventures.

2. The ability to assist physicians in their private practices so the hospital's practice enhancement programs are seen as important.

3. Continued retreats are seen as an important way to air concerns and develop alternatives.

4. There is likely to be considerable managed care growth, and the hospital and its physicians will need to be major players in these activities.

5. Some observers felt a need to improve the timeliness and responsiveness of decision making in order to meet future challenges.

SUTTER COMMUNITY HOSPITALS
(Sutter Memorial, Sutter General—common medical staff)

LOCATION: Sacramento, California

OWNERSHIP: Not-for-profit system member (Sutter Health System)

SIZE: 1220 beds (Sacramento area)

OCCUPANCY: 83 percent

KEY SERVICES: Broad range of services including neurosurgery, obstetrics, orthopedics, cardiology, cancer, psychiatry, outpatient surgery centers, mobile diagnostic imaging

---

Hospital Background and History

Sutter Health is a broad-ranging health care system comprising 12 acute care hospitals, 4 nursing centers, an Alzheimer's treatment center, and a medical research foundation, among other entities. It started as a single doctor-owned hospital in 1923, and its acute care hospital capacity has since grown to 1,220 beds. Its two primary general acute care hospitals in the Sacramento area are Sutter Memorial and Sutter General, which exist under common medical staff and governance structures as Sutter Community Hospitals. In addition to the above entities, Sutter Health has a network of immediate care centers, outpatient surgery centers, and mobile diagnostic imaging and is planning to build several integrated medical campuses. Sutter Community Hospitals is particularly strong in neurosurgery, obstetrics, orthopedics, cardiac care (including transplant), cancer care, and psychiatry.

A key event in the organization's history occurred in 1979 when a leading anesthesiologist was indicated on a morals charge. This resulted in the Joint Commission on Accreditation of Hospitals temporarily removing the accreditation status of both of Sutter's Sacramento area hospitals. Many observers feel that this event underscored the relative lack of board and management leadership at Sutter over a period of several years. The medical staff and board were so embarrassed by the situation that when a new CEO took over in 1980, the hospital vowed to commit itself to the highest possible standards of quality of care and to running a high-quality institution. Working with the board and medical staff leadership, the new CEO established a strategic planning process, resulting in the institution's first strategic plan, which provides overall direction and guidance to this day. The plan is updated annually.

Local Environment and Performance

Sutter's primary competition is the Kaiser Health Plan. Over 60 percent of the Sacramento market is involved in managed care—the majority with Kaiser. In order to compete, Sutter is a 28-percent owner of Foundation Health, Inc., the next largest HMO in the Sacramento area with 180,000 enrollees. The relationship with Foundation Health has placed some stress on the hospital-physician relationship because most physicians do not believe Foundation compensates fairly. In addition to the local HMO and managed care pressures, Sutter and its physicians also feel the pressures of the DRGs, California's MediCal reimbursement rates, and a competitive managed care/preferred provider environment in the commercial insurance sector.

Sutter is doing well financially and is generally acknowledged as the market leader. From 1985 through 1989 the occupancy rate at its hospitals averaged 83 percent. Inpatient admissions increased somewhat, while outpatients visits increased by about 23 percent. The hospital's operating margin declined from 10.1 percent in 1985 to 6.1 percent in 1989, but its total profit margin held constant at 8.4 percent.

Management Stability

Since 1980, Sutter Health has enjoyed good management stability. The current CEO has been with Sutter for 10 years. Most physician leaders have been associated with Sutter between 10 and 25 years. The newest member of the management team is the vice president for health systems development, who has been present for nearly 3 years.

Medical Staff Organization and Physician Involvement

There are 903 staff members at Sutter's Sacramento hospitals of whom 78 percent are board certified; most have overlapping practices with one or more Mercy Hospitals in the area. Approximately 61 percent practice either as solo practitioners or in two- or three-person partnerships, while 32 percent are in groups of six or more physicians.

The chief of staff and vice chief serve two-year terms. The chief is paid a $20,000 stipend by the medical staff. There are 4 physician voting members on the hospital's 16-member governing board including the chief of staff and vice chief. The CEO and COO are also members of the governing board with voting privileges. The CEO also participates as a voting member of the medical staff executive committee. Governing board members attend meetings of the medical staff executive committee, credentials committee, quality assurance committee, or utilization review committee upon invitation only. There is 1 physician on Sutter's 7-member holding company board. Physicians are also heavily involved in strategic planning—about 15 physicians in addition to the medical executive committee.

The hospital has a full-time paid medical director. The hospital sponsors an HMO, has an IPA, has a joint physician-hospital organization, and is involved in a number of economic joint ventures, including outpatient surgery centers and diagnostic imaging centers in addition to plans for the integrated medical campuses.

Significant Accomplishments

The most frequently mentioned significant accomplishments growing out of the hospital-physician relationship at Sutter are the following:

1. developing successful joint ventures in the areas of outpatient surgery and diagnostic imaging
2. starting several successful new clinical programs in such areas as cancer, diabetes, psychiatry, and heart transplantation
3. confronting the problems of emergency room coverage. A task force has been appointed to deal with the issue and to develop specialty call lists.
4. developing stronger physician leadership through conferences, retreats, and educational sessions
5. successfully managing four group practices and one IPA
6. the potential promise of the integrated medical campus idea

Significant Problems and Challenges

Among the most frequently reported challenges and problems facing Sutter are the following:

1. the earlier mentioned problem in staffing the emergency room. While a task force is currently addressing the problem, it is an issue that has received a lot of attention and concern on the part of the medical staff.
2. the tendency for administration, at times, to make plans without sufficient physician input. However, it was noted that when

this occurs the hospital tends to recognize it and modify its course.

3. some people's perception that Foundation Health, Inc., is poorly managed

4. dealing with the cardiovascular surgeons' desire to form a separate department. The request to have separate representation on the medical staff executive committee was turned down by the staff. The issue has temporarily subsided.

5. creation of a new medical staff category to assure quality of physicians without admitting privileges who staff Sutter's network or urgent care centers. This idea upset some physicians, and so the solution has been to create an ambulatory medicine subsection under family practice.

6. several concerns that are surfacing regarding the integrated medical campus concept, particularly in regard to who might be the most appropriate joint venture partners for implementation

Keys to the Future

In general, most respondents believe the relationship will get stronger in the future because of the challenges that it faces. Among the specifics mentioned most frequently are the following:

1. the need to develop a strong managed care model, a key to both the system's and the doctors' future success

2. the outcome of the integrated medical campus idea. It is recognized that there is need for heavy physician involvement in this process.

3. the ability to develop economically advantageous joint ventures

4. an immediate need to solve the emergency room staffing issue. Otherwise, in the words of one respondent, "It will create havoc."

5. the need to see how successful the new heart transplant program proves to be

TUCSON MEDICAL CENTER

LOCATION: Tucson, Arizona

OWNERSHIP: Not-for-profit independent, medical school affiliated

SIZE: 615 beds

OCCUPANCY: 63 percent

KEY SERVICES: Broad range of primary, secondary, and tertiary care including lithotripsy, MRI, trauma center, family care center network

---

Hospital Background and History

Tucson Medical Center, founded in 1944, offers a broad range of tertiary, secondary, and primary care services and has teaching affiliations with the University of Arizona Medical Center and Kino Community Hospital. Among its services are lithotripsy, magnetic resonance imaging, and a trauma program, in addition to a network of family care centers. Tucson Medical Center has a long history of physician involvement and is strongly involved in the Tucson community.

Local Environment and Performance

Tucson Medical Center (TMC) is perceived as one of the leading hospitals in the area. The environment is moderately competitive among the hospitals, with strong competition coming from a growing number of HMOs and PPOs. The hospital and its physicians are currently working out ways to best negotiate the managed care relationships to mutual benefit. The hospital is also examining its freestanding status to see if there are advantages to joining a system in terms of being better able to deal with managed care issues or other possible advantages.

Over the past four years (1985–1988), the hospital's occupancy has averaged 63 percent. Its inpatient admissions have held steady at around 29,000, and its outpatient visits increased approximately 28 percent. Reflecting the growing power of the purchasers, the hospital's operating margin declined from 4 percent in 1985 to break-even status in 1987, but rebounded to a positive 4.0 percent margin in 1988. Its total net margin declined from 5.1 percent in 1985 to a 0.2 percent loss in 1987, but rebounded to a positive 3.7 percent margin in 1988.

Management Stability

Tucson Medical Center has enjoyed considerable management stability over the years. Its current CEO has been the CEO of the hospital for 22 years, and the chief operating officer has been at TMC for 16 years. Many physician leaders have been associated with the institution for 15 to 20 years. A new vice president for nursing has recently been recruited.

Medical Staff Organization and Physician Involvement

Tucson Medical Center has 428 active staff physicians, of whom 90 percent are board certified and 100 percent practice at two or more hospitals in the area. Approximately 40 percent of physicians are in solo practice, and an additional 25 percent are in two- or three-person partnerships. However, approximately 15 percent of the active staff practice in groups of 16 or more physicians. The hospital has a full-time paid medical director and a full-time physician who serves as vice president for strategic planning. There are no full-time or part-time paid section chiefs. The president of the staff serves as a voting member of the hospital's seventeen-member board along with three other physicians. The chief of staff elect serves as a nonvoting member. The hospital CEO and COO are also voting members of the governing board. The holding company board is composed of nine members, of whom one is a physician. The medical staff organization's president and president elect serve two-year terms of office. Members of the hospital's governing board attend the medical staff executive committee meeting, as does the chief operating officer. The chief operating officer attends the medical staff credentials committee meeting but not the quality assurance or utilization review committee meetings. The hospital presently has no formal strategic planning committee. Most of the strategic planning and analysis activities are conducted through a joint physician-hospital organization.

The hospital has a relationship with an independent practice association, Southern Arizona Independent Physicians (SAIP), and is involved in HMO and PPO sponsorship. The hospital and SAIP also jointly own a physician-hospital organization. That organization is involved in several joint ventures including family care centers.

Significant Accomplishments

The most frequently reported accomplishments growing out of the hospital-physician relationship at Tucson are the following:

1. the development of the joint physician-hospital organization, which provides a forum for both groups to discuss issues of mutual interest

2. the development of the Southern Arizona Independent Physicians Corporation
3. the purchase of new technology, including a lithotripter and laser, and the expansion and upgrading of oncology services
4. recruitment of specialty physicians in such areas as perinatalogy and trauma surgery
5. resolving the malpractice premium issue

Significant Problems and Challenges

The most frequently reported challenges facing the hospital-physician relationship at TMC are the following:

1. the potential conflict between SAIP and the medical staff over new program development and membership criteria. SAIP emphasizes cost-effectiveness criteria that some medical staff members cannot meet. SAIP may also be involved in the development of certain programs and services such as senior care that are not available to the rest of the medical staff. This may be perceived by the rest of the staff as giving SAIP physicians an unfair competitive advantage.
2. coverage for the emergency room trauma services. Neurosurgeons and orthopedists have recently complained about encroachment on their time from treating patients in the trauma area.
3. managing contract care relationships with the various HMOs including decisions regarding who to include and who not to include and when to drop various carriers
4. physicians' perceptions of the need to make quicker decisions and to follow through with these decisions. Recently an ENT group left the hospital campus; many physicians believe that was due to a delay in decision making.
5. improving physician-nurse relationships. Some physicians perceive problems with nursing practice at the hospital.

Keys to the Future

Among the more frequently mentioned items holding important implications for the future of the hospital-physician relationship at TMC are the following:

1. how well the hospital and physicians do in regard to managed care. Can the PHO be used to develop mutually beneficial ar-

rangements? Mechanisms must be found to tie the physician closer to the hospital.

2. how well the current discussions and possible outcomes of a merger with Samaritan Health Services are handled. Such a merger, were it to occur, would create understandable anxieties on the part of some physicians, and these will have to be managed carefully.

3. the need to further strengthen the referral system from outlying areas. There is a need to develop a broader based primary care network in a way that is acceptable to specialty physicians.

4. the need for continuing success with joint venture activities.

WEST ALLIS MEMORIAL

LOCATION: West Allis, Wisconsin

OWNERSHIP: Not-for-profit independent

SIZE: 238 beds

OCCUPANCY: 69 percent

KEY SERVICES: Basic primary and secondary care and selected tertiary care, MRI

Hospital Background and History

West Allis is a 238-bed community hospital located in West Allis, Wisconsin. It was built by the city in 1961, and the town council appointed the first board. The key event in the hospital's history was a major conflict in the late 1960s between the medical staff, on the one hand, and the CEO and board on the other. The medical staff felt the hospital needed to add more services and new technology (for example, the hospital did not have an emergency room); the CEO and board disagreed. A series of lawsuits were brought against the hospital resulting in a temporary loss of admissions, the resignation of the CEO, and mass resignations on the part of board members. The new 13-member board was appointed in 1970 along with a new CEO. A new board and CEO immediately developed a close relationship with the physicians who were strongly committed to the hospital and to the community. The hospital provides basic primary and secondary care services and selected tertiary care services. It has a reputation as a very fine community hospital attached to a larger metropolitan market.

Local Environment and Performance

West Allis operates in a moderately competitive environment. Economic viability issues are growing in importance for both the hospital and physicians. The issues are primarily centered around relationships with managed care providers. The hospital was among the first hospitals in the state to start a PPO in 1983, although it is not currently operational. The hospital and its physicians have also had varying relationships with HMOs. In order to better position themselves for the future, the hospital entered into discussions with three other hospitals in the area regarding possible merger, consolidation, or affiliation. At this time, they have decided against such an arrangement.

The hospital has done well in its increasingly competitive environment. Inpatient occupancy has averaged 69 percent over the past four years. Inpatient admissions have grown slightly, as have outpatient visits. The hospital's operating margin has been between 3 and 4 percent over the 1985–1988 period, as has its total net margin.

Management Stability

West Allis enjoys considerable management stability. The current CEO has been in the position for 18 years, and the chairman of the hospital's boards for 15 years. The vice president for nursing has been at the institution for over 20 years. Most of the physician leaders have been with the hospital from its inception.

Medical Staff Organization and Physician Involvement

West Allis has an active staff of 148 physicians, of whom 98 percent are board certified and 95 percent have appointments at one or more other hospitals in the area. However, a nucleus of approximately 75 to 100 physicians admit primarily to West Allis. Ninety-eight percent of the physicians' practices are solo or small partnerships and groups of no more than five physicians.

The president and president elect of the staff serve two-year terms. There is no executive vice president, medical director, or any paid full-time or part-time section chiefs. There are three voting physician members on the hospital's thirteen member board. These are appointed by the board. In addition, four physicians are actively involved in the hospital's strategic planning committee. The board has its own quality assurance committee to whom the physicians make a report. The CEO is not a member of the governing board. The CEO, senior vice president for operations, and senior vice president for nursing are active, but not voting, participants in the medical executive committee. The CEO also regularly attends the credentials committee meeting of the medical staff. The hospital has an IPA and is involved in HMO discounts.

Significant Accomplishments

Among the most significant accomplishments growing out of the hospital-physician relationship at West Allis over the past year or two are the following:

1. surviving the changes involving managed care relationships without major negative incidents

2. purchasing equipment for the urologists, an MRI scanner plus expansion of the hospital's operating room, and state-of-the-art technology in all installations

3. working constantly to improve the ability of physicians to practice. This is done through public relations, a referral service, community outreach, and related activities.

4. successful recruitment of new physicians through a primary care clinic

5. building a physician office building

Significant Problems and Challenges

Among the most frequently reported challenges and problems facing the hospital and its physicians over the past year or two are the following:

1. working through the possible four-hospital merger. Ongoing discussions involve 12 key leaders including 4 physicians.

2. the challenges of dealing with managed care relationships

3. disagreements over what physicians should be on the hospital referral list

4. recruiting new physicians in family practice and internal medicine

Keys to the Future

Among the factors most frequently reported as holding keys to the future successful evolution of the hospital-physician relationship at West Allis are the following:

1. handling of the four-hospital merger

2. handling of the managed care issue

3. the need for continued strong medical staff leadership and the need to maintain mutual respect

4. the general impression that relationships may become somewhat more strained and less cohesive in the near future and, thus, require continued communication and involvement of all parties

Index

About the Author

Stephen M. Shortell is the A. C. Buehler Distinguished Professor of Hospital and Health Services Management and Professor of Organization Behavior at the J. L. Kellogg Graduate School of Management, Northwestern University. He also holds appointments in the Medical School and the Department of Sociology and is Director of the Program on Organization Behavior in Health at the University's Center for Health Services and Policy Research. Shortell received his B.B.A. from the University of Notre Dame; his M.P.H. from the University of California, Los Angeles; and his M.B.A. and Ph.D. in the Behavioral Sciences from the Graduate School of Business, University of Chicago. He taught at the University of Chicago and the University of Washington before joining the Northwestern faculty in 1982.

Shortell's main interests in recent years have been studying the performance of health care organizations, exploring the processes associated with strategic adaptation, and examining the relationship between professionals and organizations. He has published extensively in these and related areas. His most recent book (with Ellen Morrison and Bernard Friedman), *Strategic Choices for America's Hospitals: Managing Change in Turbulent Times,* received the George R. Terry Book of the Year Award from the Academy of Management. Among his previous books are *Hospital-Physician Joint Ventures: A National Demonstration in Primary Care* (1984, with Thomas M. Wickizer and John R. C. Wheeler) and *Health Care Management: A Text in Organization Theory and Behavior* (2d ed., 1988, with Arnold D. Kaluzny). He is the recipient of the 1986 Dean Conley Article of the Year Award from the American College of Healthcare Executives for his article "The Medical Staff of the Future: Replanting the Garden" (published in *Frontiers of Health Services Management,* Fall 1985); and the 1990 Edgar C. Hayhow Award for his article (with Ellen Morrison and

Susan Hughes) "The Keys to Successful Diversification: Lessons from Leading Hospital Systems" (published in *Hospital and Health Services Administration*, Winter 1989).

Shortell has been a visiting lecturer and fellow at several universities; is a frequent presenter at academic and professional meetings; has served on the editorial boards of several professionals journals, including *The Academy of Management Review, The Academy of Management Journal, Health Services Research, Medical Care*, and *The Journal of Health and Social Behavior*; and is an adviser and consultant to many private and public organizations. He is a member of the Institute of Medicine of the National Academy of Sciences, and has served as president of the Association for Health Services Research and as chairman of the Accrediting Commission for Graduate Education in Health Services Administration.